They Were Still Born

They Were Still Born

Personal Stories about Stillbirth

Edited by
Janel C. Atlas

With a foreword by
Elizabeth McCracken

ROWMAN & LITTLEFIELD PUBLISHERS, INC.
Lanham • Boulder • New York • Toronto • Plymouth, UK

Published by Rowman & Littlefield Publishers, Inc.
A wholly owned subsidiary of The Rowman & Littlefield Publishing Group, Inc.
4501 Forbes Boulevard, Suite 200, Lanham, Maryland 20706
http://www.rowmanlittlefield.com

Estover Road, Plymouth PL6 7PY, United Kingdom

British Library Cataloguing in Publication Information Available

Library of Congress Cataloging-in-Publication Data

They were still born : personal stories about stillbirth / edited by Janel C. Atlas.
p. cm.
Includes bibliographical references and index.
ISBN 978-1-4422-0412-6 (cloth : alk. paper) — ISBN 978-1-4422-0414-0 (electronic)
1. Stillbirth—Popular works. I. Atlas, Janel C., 1982–
RG631.T44 2010
618.3'2—dc22 2010020807

™ The paper used in this publication meets the minimum requirements of American National Standard for Information Sciences—Permanence of Paper for Printed Library Materials, ANSI/NISO Z39.48-1992.

Printed in the United States of America

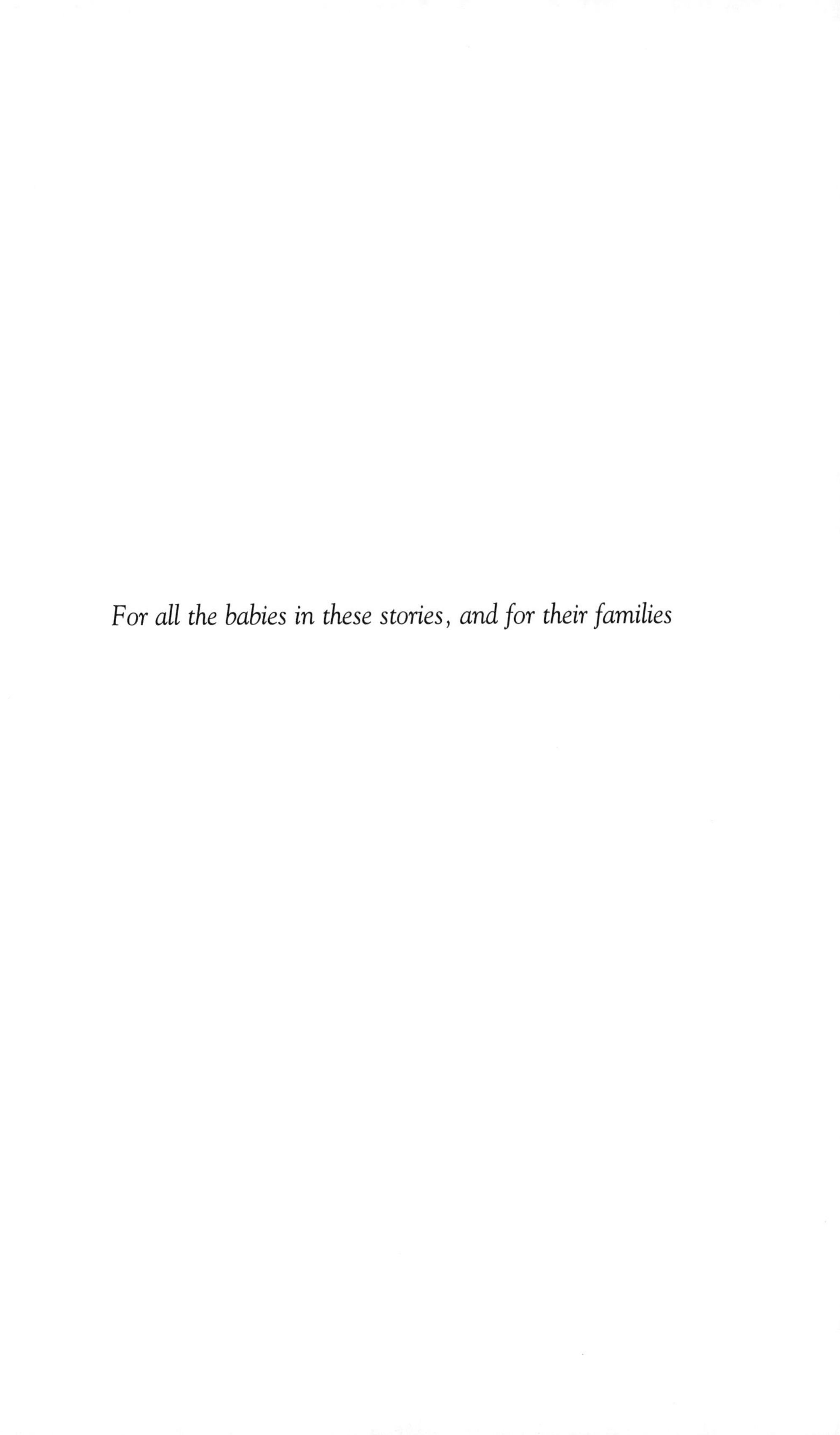

For all the babies in these stories, and for their families

Contents

Acknowledgments xi

Foreword xiii
Elizabeth McCracken

Introduction xvii
Janel C. Atlas

Part I: They Were Still Born: Personal Stories about Stillbirth

Chapter 1 What No One Tells You 1
Virginia Williams

Chapter 2 Blindsided 7
Alan Goldenbach

Chapter 3 Two Children, One Living 13
David Hlavsa

Chapter 4 The Traumatic Contradiction: When Birth and Death Collide 19
Joanne Cacciatore

Chapter 5 Living with (and without) Caleb 29
Kelley Krahling

Chapter 6 He Changed Our World 37
Marion J. Flores

Chapter 7 Mothering Grief 45
Angie M. Yingst

Chapter 8 In a Wild Place 51
Rachel Graham

Chapter 9 Born, Again 57
Meng Kiat Tan

Chapter 10 Just One Family 65
Jenell Williams Paris

Chapter 11 "Then Comes the Baby in the Baby Carriage" 71
Sherokee Ilse

Chapter 12 A Plan Gone Awry 81
Monica Murphy LeMoine

Chapter 13 Saying "Grace": Family's and Friends' Responses to My Daughter's Stillbirth 87
Candy McVicar

Chapter 14 Our Christmas Angel 95
Laura Villmer

Chapter 15 She Was Significant 103
Nina Bennett

Chapter 16 How Death Can Bring Life: A Caregiver's Perspective 109
Kathleen Skipper

Chapter 17 Invincible No More: What My Daughter's Stillbirth Taught Me about Life 119
Tim Nelson

Chapter 18 Reunion Group 125
Amy L. Abbey

Chapter 19 Standing in the Shadows of Grief 135
Janel C. Atlas

Chapter 20 Grief and Creativity 141
Kara L. C. Jones

Chapter 21 The Year of Angels 151
Suzanne Pullen

Part II: The Way Forward
Edited by Janel C. Atlas, Sherokee Ilse, and Suzanne Pullen

Chapter 22 Honoring and Remembering Your Baby 173
Janel C. Atlas

Chapter 23 Creative Expressions of Grief 181
Kara L. C. Jones

Chapter 24 What We Know about Stillbirth 185
Ruth Fretts, MD, MPH

Chapter 25 Emerging Research 199
Janel C. Atlas

Resources 217

Notes 227

Bibliography 233

Index 239

About the Contributors 247

Acknowledgments

This book is the result of many, many people's work and support, and it never could have come to fruition without the amazing people who were on board from the very beginning: Nina Bennett, who encouraged me to pitch the idea to editor after editor; Dr. Crystal Downing, the best writing teacher I've ever had; Joanne Cacciatore and Sherokee Ilse, both of whom helped me before they even knew me; John Micklos, for his encouragement and editor's wisdom for my book proposal and essay; Suzanne Pullen, for her enthusiasm and intelligent coordination of multiple projects all at once; and my supportive family and friends, especially Janet Brown, Denice Grawe, and Heather Suchanec-Cooper, who were with me through the dark days after my loss and gave me the courage to speak Beatrice's name aloud.

I want to acknowledge the emotionally difficult work the contributors did, and their fearless delving into the intensely private and personal stories they have lived. And this book would not be in your hands were it not for Suzanne Staszak-Silva at Rowman & Littlefield, who saw the need for this collection and championed it.

Last, I want to thank my wonderful husband and two sweet (living) daughters for their patience, support, and love as I've wrangled chapters and rewritten sections and pulled this whole thing together. And I thank Beatrice, my little Bea, for giving me her story and for making a difference in the lives of so many.

Foreword

Elizabeth McCracken, *author of* An Exact Replica of a Figment of My Imagination

In the end, the stories are mostly what we have left of our children.

Nearly the moment I learned he was dead, I knew I would write about my first child. We were still in the first hospital, where he would have been delivered had he lived; soon we would get in our car and drive to the second hospital, which for some obscure reason (money, I think—it must have been money) was better for delivering a dead child. The strangers who looked at me sobbing, clinging to my husband, would have thought me anything but detached. But part of me had broken off, had walked up the stairs to some brain garret, shut the door, and sat down to record. Perhaps that's why the first day is still so clear to me, while I see the later days as shadows through a frosted window. Through tears, I guess I mean. Bad habit, good habit, I don't know—but I was converting what happened into sentences already. The horror was indescribable, so I would try to describe it. Nonsensical, so I needed to make sense of it.

I felt like I needed to write my own story so that I could read it and understand what it meant.

Then the second day—the baby was dead but I hadn't delivered him—a friend of mine told me that there was an essay in the *New Yorker* that very week about, as she put it, "the same thing." And that stopped my sentence making. I'm not sure why. Maybe because in those first days when I believed many things that weren't true—that I would prefer not to see my dead son, that there was no way in the world that I would ever be happy again—I believed that there could only be one thing written on the subject. At any rate, that was the moment I began to really think about what had happened to me, not about how I would relate the story to someone else.

Then in the fall I was pregnant again and could not write much of anything.

And then that son was born, alive, skinny, healthy, handsome, and I found I needed to write—or go crazy. Not for publication. Notes for something else. At the end of three weeks, though, I seemed to have a book. Writing it had saved my sanity.

But that wasn't the only piece of important writing I'd done during Gus's first summer. A friend came to meet him. Her stepdaughter had recently had her first baby, but the sad thing was, her best friend's first baby, due at the same time, died, full-term. This was the first baby I knew of who died after mine did. "Give me her e-mail address," I demanded. My friend said, "I'll ask."

I think I demanded this stranger's e-mail address several more times until I finally got it, and then I wrote to the stranger, whose name was Lena. It took a while before she wrote me back. And then we wrote more often. And here was the thing that I hadn't understood about other women's stories: Lena told me what had happened to her first son, Strick, and I could think, plainly, *Well, that's the worst thing I've heard of. That is too sad to bear.*

And that realization made me a little more tender with myself. I had already finished my memoir when we started our correspondence, and I had decided not to spend a great deal of time rewriting it: it was an accurate portrait of how I felt three to six weeks after the birth of my second child, about a year after the death of my first. I felt I had already gotten everything I could out of writing it.

But writing to Lena was just as important to me. There had been moments over the past year when I was not sure that I would survive. I don't mean literally; I wasn't suicidal, and I didn't think I would die of grief, even if occasionally I wished I could lapse into a grief-induced coma. I mean, I thought for the rest of my life I would be a fearful, grief-stricken person, of no use to anyone. Writing to Lena, reading her e-mails, I understood that I had survived and that she would, too.

That, I think, is what other people's stories can do. You understand that they, like you, went through something terrible; you see that they, like you, will survive it.

Lena had her second child—a second son, another thing we had in common—about fourteen months later. And I happened to be flying to her city shortly afterward, and I still remember holding that little baby (about six pounds at birth, just like Gus was) and thinking about what she had written to me— that when this baby was born, he was "filled with heavenly light"—and I knew it was a simple fact. And Lena herself, and Geoff, her husband—it really was like meeting family. We were related.

When I told some memoir-writing friends about my plans for publishing the book, they said, "Get ready for every sad story in the world to land in your mailbox." They said how exhausting it could be, listening to and reading over other people's sad stories. But that's the thing about losing a child to stillbirth: our stories are all more similar than they are different. I suspect that the loss of a spouse is as various as the spouses themselves. Ditto the loss of a grown child or a best friend. Those of us who have lost children at birth or just before or just after are a more closely related family, I think, both because of the nature of the loss, and how little the loss is spoken of by people who haven't been through it. I do get e-mails and letters from women and men who have lost children, and I'm grateful. You can't do anything for a stillborn child except know and acknowledge that he or she existed. We have nothing to give each other but our stories.

Here is a book of stories, a book of children: every one particular, every one—if you have been through it or know someone who has—horribly familiar. They are all beautiful. They have all been made with love.

They will be of great use to you.

Introduction

Janel C. Atlas

Childbirth should be a time of joy, of excitement, of meeting a long-awaited infant and introducing him or her to the world. The bustle of activity in the delivery room. The glint of shiny balloons with cheery welcomes. The satisfaction of cuddling a new baby, naming your baby, and going home with dreams for the life you'll have as a parent.

When a baby dies before birth, the experience of labor and delivery could not be more different. It slows down, becomes a shadowy pantomime. For parents whose baby dies during labor, it can be truly terrifying, with attempts at speeding the baby's delivery and efforts at resuscitation.

However a baby is stillborn—whether a problem was diagnosed earlier in the pregnancy or the loss is completely unforeseen, whether at 20 weeks' or 42 weeks' gestation, whether an answer is ever found for why the baby died—that baby was *still* born. That baby still has parents, grandparents, and family members who know of his or her existence, who miss the baby, and who cannot understand why the baby couldn't stay.

The silence of birthing my stillborn baby shattered me. Up until a week before, at my 35-week doctor's appointment, everything in this, my second pregnancy, had gone according to plan: the gloriously obvious positive home pregnancy test, the sound of a happy little heartbeat, the growing belly, and the plans for what this baby would be like and what she would bring to our lives.

But without warning, my storybook pregnancy ended with a baby born still, her life ended before she even left my body.

I had no idea what to do, so my husband and I went with our instincts. We called family and friends, asked our pastor to come bless her body, and spent several hours with our daughter. We tried to memorize her features; my husband lifted her eyelid to discover that her eyes were brown, like her sister's.

And then we left the hospital. Drove home. Tried to live.

Stillbirth, defined as the death of an infant between 20 weeks' gestation and birth, is a tragedy repeated four million times per year worldwide. In America, nearly thirty thousand babies are stillborn each year. These thousands of mothers feel their babies slip silently from their bodies, the only sound in the delivery room their own sobs. Like my husband and I did, each mother and father must go home and mourn the death of a child who will never breathe, gurgle, learn to walk, or go to school.

For families struggling with the grief of having stillborn babies, the quest for answers, information, and support can prove challenging. I remember desperately searching the shelves at my local public library, praying to find a book about stillbirth. For all the books about pregnancy—eat right, the vegan way; perfect baby names; natural birthing options—there was no one book offering various perspectives on surviving a stillbirth. I read several books that helped me, but I found myself turning to online support groups and chat rooms to find stories about others' losses. I craved personal narratives by parents who had had a stillborn baby.

How did they survive it?

Would it ever get easier or hurt less?

Would trying for another baby help, or would it only make me miss my dead daughter more?

What were the chances a subsequent pregnancy would end in another life-shattering loss?

My search for a book addressing these questions ultimately led me to edit this book. I began gathering new essays from some of the best writers on the difficult topic of stillbirth. Part I consists of twenty-one essays by twenty-one contributors. Not just great writers, these contributors all know firsthand the experience of having a stillborn baby. They do not write from merely an academic or poetic perspective—they write from the dark, from the deep pain of having a baby die before he or she is even born. And yet the essays in this collection are so much more than stories about dead babies. The essays have the same starting point, but each writer shares his or her story of loss from a different angle. These stories offer hope, insight, and even humor about this topic, which is still often taboo in our society.

In "What No One Tells You," Virginia Williams explores the tumult of having to answer the question "Where's your baby?" In "Blindsided," *Washington Post* writer Alan Goldenbach describes the anger and dismay he felt at not having heard anything about rates of stillbirth. Then his son was stillborn, and Goldenbach struggled with society's pervasive silence about stillbirth.

David Hlavsa describes the differences in protocol and social expectations following the death of an older person vis-à-vis the death of a baby in "Two Children, One Living." In her chapter, "The Traumatic Contradiction," Joanne Cacciatore—MISS Foundation founder, grief specialist, and author of *Dear Cheyenne*—writes about the profound collision of birth and death.

Kelley Krahling's chapter, "Living with (and without) Caleb," depicts the early hours and days of grief and provides an intimate look at post-loss psychology. Marion Flores's "He Changed Our World" describes her long and beautiful journey to motherhood, culminating in adopting two sons after the death of her only biological child. Blogger Angie Yingst writes, "I am a modern woman with tattoos and good health insurance whose daughter was stillborn for no medical reason whatsoever." In an instant, Yingst became a mother to both the memory of her deceased baby and her very much alive two-year-old daughter; she shares her story in "Mothering Grief."

Rachel Graham looks back sixteen years to her daughter's stillbirth and reflects on the impact that loss had on her faith ("In a Wild Place"). Taking a different approach to understanding her son Ferdinand's stillbirth, Glow in the Woods blogger Meng Kiat Tan questions her maternal instincts but ends with joy in "Born, Again." Anthropologist Jenell Williams Paris juxtaposes the death of her triplets with the all-too-common incidence of stillbirth and infant loss in an impoverished Brazilian slum in "Just One Family."

Sherokee Ilse, prominent author of pregnancy and infant loss literature (including *Empty Arms*) and long-standing parent advocate, reflects back on the more than twenty-five years since her son Brennan's death in "'Then Comes the Baby in the Baby Carriage.'" Monica Murphy LeMoine, author of *Knocked Up, Knocked Down: Postcards of Miscarriage and Other Misadventures from the Brink of Parenthood*, tells a story about how the pain of losing a baby can strike at the unlikeliest moment, like on a romantic getaway weekend ("A Plan Gone Awry"). In "Saying 'Grace': Family's and Friends' Responses to My Daughter's Stillbirth," Candy McVicar shares words that gave her grief and words that gave her comfort and support.

The holidays won't ever be the same for Laura Villmer, whose daughter was stillborn on Christmas Day 2004; Villmer tells her story in "Our Christmas Angel." Nina Bennett, author of *Forgotten Tears: A Grandmother's Journey through Grief*, offers a poignant portrayal of the dual pain of stillbirth for a grandparent, both grieving the death of a much-loved baby and witnessing the pain of a grown child ("She Was Significant"). Nurse and bereavement specialist Kathleen Skipper's first son was anencephalic and lived only a few hours in 1966. In "How Death Can Bring Life: A Caregiver's Perspective," Skipper shares how her own loss led to her efforts to help newly bereaved parents face their grief and make memories with their babies in the short time they have.

Tim Nelson is the coauthor (with Sherokee Ilse) of *Couple Communication after a Baby Dies*. Nelson offers a father's perspective on showing emotion in the wake of a stillbirth in "Invincible No More: What My Daughter's Stillbirth Taught Me about Life." Long Island mother Amy Abbey ("Reunion Group") writes about what she gained from joining a support group after her son's stillbirth, and how her subsequent pregnancy inspired her to write and publish *Journeys: Stories of Pregnancy after Loss*. My contribution, "Standing in the Shadows of Grief," explores how I coped with the first year of life after my daughter was stillborn, and the light that shone in and enabled me to find happiness again.

Mother Henna blogger and artist Kara L. C. Jones imparts her wisdom in exploring the arts as a medium for grief exploration and healing in "Grief and Creativity." The final chapter in part I, "The Year of Angels," is a series of poems and letters by Suzanne Pullen, a communications instructor, lecturer, performer, and writer.

Part II consists of four chapters on "The Way Forward." In "Honoring and Remembering Your Baby," I offer a myriad of ways to parent your child's memory, gleaned from conversations with bereaved parents. Whether you seek a one-time idea or an ongoing project to do to honor your baby, this chapter provides inspiration and guidance. Kara L. C. Jones, a writer, artist, and grief coach, provides prompts for tapping into grief in healing ways in "Creative Expressions of Grief."

Dr. Ruth Fretts, an obstetrician-gynecologist at Harvard Vanguard Medical Associates and assistant professor at Harvard Medical School, wrote "What We Know about Stillbirth." She gives vital background about what stillbirth is, how and why it happens, and what to consider when embarking on a subsequent pregnancy. With the help of doctors, experts, and researchers around the world, "Emerging Research" presents what we're learning about stillbirth and stillbirth prevention. And finally, to help you sort through the many available resources out there for bereaved parents, we've put together a list of resources, which includes helpful books, websites, and organizations.

My hope, shared by all the wonderful contributors to this book, is that reading these stories and the accompanying materials will provide you with solace and the realization that you are not alone on this painful path—that others have gone before you and have found their way—and the assurance that your baby's life was and is significant. For even though your baby was stillborn, your baby was still born. You are still a parent, and you have the painful opportunity to make meaning through your baby's brief life. May the words and wisdom in this book give you, as contributor Virginia Williams eloquently puts it in her essay, not a map to follow through grief, but perspective from those who have gone before you on this journey.

PART I

THEY WERE STILL BORN: PERSONAL STORIES ABOUT STILLBIRTH

CHAPTER ONE

What No One Tells You

Virginia Williams

It would have been an innocent question in most circumstances, in the kind of world I used to believe in, where pregnancies ended happily. But when directed to me unexpectedly after a year of grieving for my son Ben, it only pointed out the loneliness of my loss and the naïveté of the questioner.

"Where's your baby?"

Without any warning or preamble on a dreary December morning, a woman I barely knew turned to me in the one place where I thought I was safe from insensitive remarks and stupid questions: in the arms of the church that had supported me and my husband as we grieved our lost child. But on this particular Sunday, a near stranger who had somehow missed the announcements, the tears, the grief heavy on our faces for the past months, asked the one question I didn't want to answer.

"Where's your baby?" she asked again as I stared at her, bewildered, not sure if I had heard her correctly. *Was she serious? How could she not know?*

My last conversation with this woman had taken place nearly 365 days earlier, in almost the exact same spot and at the same Christmas program where she cornered me now. Then, I'd been happy to tell her that I was expecting my second child, a boy, due on the third of January. Today, I wanted her to melt or vaporize—anything to get her out of my sight.

"What?" I replied, incredulous that anyone who knew me even remotely could be ignorant of what had happened to my family, the death and birth of our son on New Year's Eve morning the previous year.

Once more she repeated her question, and I stumbled out that horrendous phrase: "He's dead." You might hope that a reasonable person would stop the conversation there, hastily say, "I'm sorry," and try to discover the circumstances of the death by asking another party, but on that morning I was not to be so lucky.

"What happened?" she asked, and I told her, as quickly as I could, that my son died from a knot in his umbilical cord, pulled tight in my womb, ending his life when it had barely begun. *Where,* I wondered, *have you been for the last twelve months? How have you not noticed, in those times you must have seen us, that there was no baby in our arms?*

Sadly, this woman was not the first to ask me about the whereabouts of my child; another woman, a clerk at a local store, asked me on four separate occasions where Ben was. Once upon a time I would never have believed the absurdity of people's reactions to my child's death or their tactless comments, but losing Ben taught me much about things I never wanted to know.

My son's death is the dividing line in my life, a firm delineation between what I knew and believed about living in the world before we lost him and what life became after his death.

"Before," with a capital B, was that blissful, happy time full of plans and hopes and dreams, full of future possibilities. If you were anything like me, you read pregnancy books with tips to prepare for the coming changes and the way your body would transform itself to support a new, tiny being. You were perhaps overwhelmed by the myriad of magazines doling out advice about how your relationship with your partner would alter under the strains and joys of parenthood, while you depended on magazine articles that specified exactly how many undershirts, diapers, and pairs of tiny socks to purchase before bringing your baby home.

Everything you needed to know was there for you in print, step-by-step, month-by-month, alongside the unsolicited advice of friends, family, and strangers. Nowhere did you see, or take notice of, any mention of what could go wrong. Sure, you were aware of the risk of miscarriage in the first trimester, but after that? Wasn't it all smooth sailing until the day your baby was born? Trimesters Two and Three were easy to get through, once the danger and uncertainty of the first three months had passed and there was the promise of a new life to look forward to.

And then, near the very end, when the baby is so close you can picture him in the crib, nearly feel him in your arms, the unthinkable happens. The one thing you didn't read about in all those articles, just as it happened to me—to you—as it happens to an incomprehensible number of families every year. Your baby dies before he is even born, and everything you dreamed, everything you hoped for, shatters like a pane of glass under hurricane-force winds. There are no instructions to guide you through unrelenting grief. There is no contour map to tell you that the road ahead will be bumpy, nor how high the mountains you must climb or how low the valleys you must traverse. There is no timeline to let you know that in six months, eight months, two years, you can expect the pain to have diminished tenfold.

Despite what anyone says about the stages of grief, sorrow is not linear; it ebbs and flows each day, sometimes each hour, for as long as it needs, be that months or years. There are no road signs along grief's highway to tell you that the path ahead is slippery and full of curves, or how many miles you have to navigate before you reach your destination: the day when you smile and laugh again, when the pain no longer cripples you in all your waking moments.

In life After, none of the books you read during that time you now call Before will matter. No words written down in black and white could have readied you for the moment you discovered that your child died before he took his first breath. There is no way to prepare someone for the long months of bottomless sorrow that will fill every moment of every day. No one can describe or explain the emptiness that follows the death of your baby.

It is a sad and secretive club you've joined, vastly different from the one you anticipated entering months ago when two lines appeared on the pregnancy test, promising to permanently alter your life. Before you received your membership to this vast group, you were likely unaware that this lonely sorority of sorrow, grief, and shock existed. Most probably, in that easy, happy time you now think of as Before, you never imagined how deeply anguish could penetrate a life.

There are many things, in these early days, that no one will be there to tell you, after the condolences have stopped and the outside world has returned to normal. Neighbors and acquaintances will unknowingly visit additional heartbreak upon you when they stop you on the sidewalk or in the produce section of the grocery store to ask where your baby is—an ordinary, everyday question to ask someone they knew was pregnant, but now a question so weighted with emotion and sorrow you won't ask it of anyone ever again.

People will surreptitiously glance your way, trying to gauge how you're managing and judging your pain by appearances alone. Some will choose to tell you that they lost their pet a few months ago and therefore know just how you feel. Others will whisper behind your back, hoping that you won't notice, when you long for them to speak to you, face you, ask you how you are and say your child's name—for he had a name, and a face, and he was so close to perfect. So close to coming home. There may even be an unimaginably stupid few who ask you more than once where your baby is, and you will grit your teeth each time and recount your story, wanting nothing more than to scream, grab them and shake them, and ask why they can't remember this one thing: your baby is dead.

Other voices from Before, once echoing with advice and opinions, are silent now. Worse, well-meaning but woefully misinformed individuals will tell you it's for the best, you have an angel now, at least you hadn't started to love him yet, you can always have another. On occasion, even years later, some friend or relation will ask if you had to give birth to him, did you hold him, was he normal? *How*, you will wonder, *can people be so stupid?* but then you realize how little you knew, Before, about stillbirth. No book, no article, no well-intentioned word of warning, told you that your baby could die days before his due date, after the crib was assembled, the diapers purchased, the coming-home outfit packed in a hospital bag. No, nothing could have prepared you for this.

And now you know: you know what to say to the mothers and fathers who will come behind you—for they will come, other couples who will lose a child just like you have. You will never share your hard-earned wisdom with anyone beforehand, while they are glowing with love and joy, waiting for their miracle to be born. Now you are the angel of death to pregnant couples who know your story, and in the glow of their bliss, you sit and shake your head and think, "It could still all go wrong." Most of the time, perhaps all of the time, circumstances won't go wrong for them and you will wonder, *Why me? Why did it have to be me?* Even though you know full well it simply happened for no other reason than it could.

What no one tells you is so much more than anyone should have to know. But one day, years beyond your loss, when you have discovered how many others of us there truly are, through support groups or on the Internet, when you have sifted through the people who make thoughtless remarks, you will discover you're not alone. Individuals will step forward, quietly, to tell you about the child they have lost. Bit by bit you will discover that many others have survived the death of their baby, and eventually you will realize that you are surviving, too.

After six years I can say I have endured the worst heartbreak imaginable. There are still painful silences in my life, times when people who know full well I have three children will mention "both" my pregnancies, or, if I am feeling frustrated with parenting, suggest I imagine how I would feel if I had three children instead of two. *Ah, but I* do *have three children*, I think to myself, wanting, more than anything, for my Ben to be remembered. The ache of his loss, however, is manageable now, though I think of him every day and will forever wonder who he would have been.

Telling people about my son is far easier than I could have imagined once upon a time. Ben was here and he remains a part of my life, every day, and though I choose carefully just whom I tell about him, it no longer brings me to tears each time. Yes, life has changed irrevocably and will be forever bittersweet. My happily-ever-after is not what I'd envisioned and I have changed permanently, as anyone who loses a child does. From an awful period in my life I have gained an unexpected solidarity with others who understand—who know enough not to ask, "Where's your baby?"

If you have crossed from life Before to life After a stillbirth, you are uniquely prepared to understand, to connect with others who have also faced this tragedy. If and when someone you know, or the friend of a friend, or the couple down the street loses a child, you will know what to do, what to say. You can warn them that there will be songs they won't listen to ever again, movies that will forever serve as a reminder of a time, now very long ago and far away, full of a happiness hard to remember. When they ask you how long it will be before the pain stops, before they no longer cry every day, you can reply that, while there is no certain point in time when life is all right again, it will, one day, stop hurting so much. On that day, not soon, but sometime, they will discover themselves smiling, just a little. It takes time, you answer, the passing of each season and the marking of the first full year without the one you want, before you realize you are doing exactly this: bearing it, managing, living. Not the way you wanted to, but living just the same.

Eventually, all those things you never wanted to learn can be put to use, can serve as a warning of the path ahead for those who come along behind. When that time comes, you will be ready; you will exhibit a strength you never before imagined and reach out your hand to a parent sitting on the precipice of loss. When you are asked, you will say, "No, there is no map for you to follow. But I can tell you what I've learned."

CHAPTER TWO

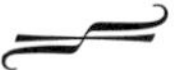

Blindsided

Alan Goldenbach

A couple of weeks after my son died the day before he was supposed to be born, I went to a large bookstore seeking reassurance.

Once inside the front door, I swallowed hard and headed immediately for the one shelf I should have avoided: the pregnancy and childbirth section. Looking at the cover of each book—the words connoting hope, the images of pregnant women and couples cradling newborns—felt like a knife twisting in my chest. Yet, I had come to the store to prove a point to myself. I wasn't turning back.

I picked up one of the featured titles, one that was facing outward and had about a dozen copies behind it, and immediately flipped to the index. I went to the S section and looked for the term *stillbirth*. There was no mention of it. I turned back a few pages to the Ms and looked under *miscarriage*, figuring maybe stillbirth was mentioned within that section.

Nothing.

I grabbed another of the popular titles and repeated my routine. No mention of stillbirth whatsoever. Two more titles left me similarly unfulfilled. Finally, I found one book, more than four hundred pages long and authored by a renowned physician, that included my target term. It described stillbirth in one paragraph on the bottom of a page (though at least it was highlighted in a gray box). It said nothing about its frequency, just that it is awful, that parents should never feel responsible for a stillbirth, and, worst of all, that 99 percent of the time the woman could have done nothing to prevent it.

I thought I might have been looking in the wrong place, so I peeked around the corner to see if the pregnancy and childbirth books extended to another shelf. They didn't.

Stillbirth, the culprit that destroys more than one in every two hundred pregnancies in this country, was glaringly absent from these books that are specifically intended to guide couples through their pregnancies, to prepare them for every possible twist or turn.

I stared briefly at the stack of books and sighed. I felt relieved. I had gotten the reassurance I sought; I didn't want to regret that my wife and I had missed something while we pored over dozens of pieces of literature during our pregnancy. As stunned as we were when our doctor told us that our son had died from a knotted umbilical cord—a fact confirmed by an autopsy—we were taken further aback by how little we knew, before our son's death, about stillbirth, its frequency, potential causes, or potential warning signs. I realized then that even had we sought out information about stillbirth in pregnancy texts, we would not have been able to find any. I began to wonder why.

A week after my visit to the bookstore, my wife and I met with her obstetrician to see if she could shed some light on our son's death. With the bookstore experience fresh in my mind, the first question I asked was why we hadn't heard anything about stillbirth. It was an even more pertinent topic, given my wife's bout with preeclampsia, which put her at an increased risk for stillbirth, as well as posing a risk to her own health. In fact, my wife had been seen weekly over the final two months of her pregnancy by a high-risk obstetrics practice to monitor the health of both her and our baby. Ultimately, though, the knotted umbilical cord that killed my son had nothing to do with my wife's preeclampsia. The latter, however, did give doctors more reason to monitor her.

Soft-spoken by nature, the obstetrician sighed, clasped her hands together and told us awkwardly from behind her desk, "Pregnancy is a happy time. Nobody wants to hear anything about something bad, much less about death."

We spent about another ninety minutes in the doctor's office, discussing my wife's health, the preeclampsia that hospitalized her for the final ten days of her pregnancy, and the dangers she would encounter if we would ever again try to get pregnant. Yet, I had a difficult time paying much attention to this other information. My mind fixated on our doctor's earlier words, seething at her betrayal of our trust.

The high-risk obstetricians never called us after our stillbirth, nor did the practice reach out to us through a letter or even an e-mail. Those doctors didn't want to discuss the one thing that they supposedly had expertise in identifying, isolating, and preventing.

My wonder about the silence that surrounds stillbirth only grew.

One in two hundred is equal to half of 1 percent. Looking to avoid that outcome, a betting man would happily take those odds. When my wife and I first learned that, our initial response was a helpless, "Well, it seems our number came up."

Consider, however, the frequency of pregnancies. Look around a large office or a church or a high school graduation. At least one person in each of those groups is going to experience a stillbirth. Remember, it's not a percentage of people, but rather, a percentage of *pregnancies* that end in a stillbirth. Most couples get pregnant more than once.

All of a sudden, one in two hundred doesn't seem so unlikely.

I did a little digging to try to learn why stillbirth, despite its alarmingly high rate of incidence in a medically advanced nation like the United States, is a shunned topic—not only in doctors' offices, but in general discourse. I was voracious in my reading and my phone calls, treating it almost as a part-time job. I remember being on the phone with a doctor while I was at an airport waiting for a flight to depart, scribbling down every statistic and detail she told me before hurrying to board the plane. Another researcher called me while I was driving, and I sat on the shoulder of a highway talking to him for a good half-hour. There was never a time nor a place when I didn't want to learn more about stillbirth.

I couldn't figure out why the general public didn't show even a passing concern. It couldn't be because stillbirth is such an awful occurrence; our country doesn't seem to have difficulty discussing and fighting to lower the rates of SIDS, Down syndrome, or even AIDS. Yet, there are ten times the number of stillbirths annually in the United States compared to deaths attributed to SIDS, which has been identified as a key public health issue. I remember going furniture shopping during our pregnancy and my wife and I listening to salespeople describe crib safety features to minimize the risk of SIDS.

Prenatal testing has almost become ritual for Down syndrome—yet stillbirths occur four times as often. In fact, domestic stillbirths occur more than 2½ times as frequently as Americans succumbing to AIDS annually. I know nearly every American adult has heard of AIDS and most can discuss it openly. So why not stillbirth?

Our obstetrician told my wife and me that nothing could have been done to prevent our stillbirth. Not by us. Not by her and her five colleagues in their medical practice, each of whom we met during our pregnancy. That still didn't excuse the egregious omission of any mention of stillbirth—not before we became pregnant, when we met with her to discuss our plans, not during the pregnancy, and certainly not when my wife was hospitalized with preeclampsia. I found it impossible to accept a nonexplanation as fact simply because the supposed experts did not have an answer for its occurrence. These people became experts for precisely the opposite reason: they weren't satisfied with the status quo and their curiosity led them to find answers.

Unfortunately, I learned that my wife and I weren't the only ones being fed this line.

Dr. Ruth C. Fretts is among the handful of medical professionals who don't believe parents of stillborn children should have to accept the nonanswer answer. Fretts is an assistant professor of obstetrics and gynecology at Harvard Medical School and chair of the scientific committee for the International Stillbirth Alliance, a nonprofit collaborative that seeks to increase the understanding and prevention of stillbirth. Fretts researched the causes of fetal death at various stages of development, and she found the leading *reported* cause after 28 weeks' gestation is an unexplained cause. She found other roots of fetal death, including malnutrition and placental abruption; neither those nor any other were as common as a doctor telling a sobbing couple, "I can't tell you why this happened." I didn't take comfort in the fact that at least I know why my son died, while thousands of other couples never get an answer. In fact, this made me angrier.

Fretts said there is frustration within the medical community over its inability to reduce the rate of stillbirth, but that sentiment has fostered a sense of surrender among most doctors. Grieving parents want answers as to why their babies died, and, I, in particular, also wanted to know why we had not discussed the possibility of this prior to his death. This silence on such a common pregnancy outcome led to us being blindsided when it happened to us. The medical community pushes back, replying, "We can't do anything to prevent it, so why should we bother talking about it?"

While Fretts agreed with me that one in two hundred is far too high a number of stillbirths for a nation as medically and technologically advanced as the United States, she also pointed out why doctors are reluctant to speak about it: what about the other 199 who are going to deliver healthy babies? We'd be scaring a whole lot of people by telling them about their worst fears. I tried to put myself in that situation— being pregnant and hearing that there's a half-percent chance my greatest fear would be realized. Would I consider that fair warning or a scare tactic? Then I tried thinking about millions of other couples. Do they want to spend nine months wondering if they are destined to be like my wife and me, have their number called, and their baby will be the one in two hundred?

My biggest regret about that conversation with our obstetrician was not thinking quickly enough as I sat in her office. When she told us that parents don't want to hear about anything bad during their pregnancy, I should have countered, "Then why did you have us perform a test to see if our baby had an increased chance of being born with Down syndrome? What if that test had come back positive?"

The reason such a test is administered is that, as Fretts told me, the Down syndrome community brought the condition into public discourse. They made it a key issue for those researching fetal health and development. The community of those who lost a baby to SIDS did the same thing. They began talking about how horrible and devastating it was to endure a pregnancy, deliver and bring home a baby, and have him die suddenly and mysteriously one night. Doctors at the time were baffled; how could a baby sleeping comfortably in a crib just die, seemingly out of the blue, especially when there were no visible contributing factors? (Sounds an awful lot like stillbirth, doesn't it?)

What happened was that people started talking about their experiences, as difficult as that was, and the awkwardness of listening to their stories slowly disappeared. When these stories began to mount in number, researchers collected and analyzed data. Patterns emerged from the stories. Before you knew it, advocacy groups had sponsored major public health initiatives and education campaigns, soft mattresses and blankets vanished from cribs, and caregivers stopped putting babies to sleep on their bellies. Lo and behold, the rate of SIDS began a precipitous decline.

The medical community has identified a myriad of arbitrary factors as the most important risks to avoid for a healthy pregnancy. My wife still shakes her head at the fact that she was repeatedly warned not to eat tuna during her pregnancy because of the trace amounts of mercury present. Yet, she was never prescribed monitoring kick counts during her final trimester. When she asked one of our doctors about the importance of sleeping on her side, she was told it's important, but not critical (she slept on her side, anyway).

Research, on the other hand, had determined otherwise. A woman sleeping on her side does improve fetal health. Kick counts, too, have shown to be an accurate gauge of fetal activity and well-being.

Ultimately, what happened with SIDS is what needs to happen to reduce the rate of stillbirth. It begins with a grassroots effort. People talking and sharing their experiences will make others aware of the prevalence of stillbirths. It will also allow them to take comfort, however slight that may be, in the fact that they are part of an unfortunate but large community that, individually, feels isolated because of our society's unwillingness to embrace the gravity of stillbirths' frequency.

When that community of families assembles with one voice and pools its message (and its data), the medical community can then examine all these cases and begin to find some patterns. Those patterns can then provide the basis for new guidelines, ones that are given to every couple at the beginning of a pregnancy.

It won't eliminate stillbirths. It will scare plenty of parents whose babies are ultimately born healthy, but it would enhance their joy and give them a greater appreciation upon their babies' delivery. It would also prevent the unfortunate couples from being completely blindsided when their baby is stillborn. Trust me—not knowing is not worth the risk.

CHAPTER THREE

Two Children, One Living

David Hlavsa

When my father, who was just short of his seventy-sixth birthday, was killed in a car accident near my parents' home in upstate New York in the fall of 2007, nothing was easy, exactly. I flew in from Seattle the next morning and, as methodically as I could, began the daunting process of helping my mother make arrangements: planning his funeral, settling his estate, sorting his things. Not easy to do, but at least it wasn't hard to figure out what had to be done. However sudden a death in the family may be, there are rituals to follow, and a linear progression of tasks. The first thing is to let people know. I sat with my mother flipping through my parents' Rolodex, calling family and friends. However painful and awkward it may be to deliver such news, at least there is a script to follow. You tell them you have bad news; you tell them what happened; they say, "I'm so sorry"; and you say, "Thank you." They send flowers. They bring food. They put on sober costumes and they donate to a designated charity. They offer a handshake or an embrace and ask, in low tones, if there's anything they can do. At the memorial service, they gather to remember, to pay tribute, to comfort. But also, they gather to send the family on their way—the dead to the earth, or to the next life; the living to adjust to their new lives as best they can.

Like love, grief comes upon us; it happens to us. As with any force that acts on us, we may resist it or we may surrender to it, but either way it changes us and it changes everything around us. The rituals of bereavement, the very roteness of the prescribed activities, help us to recognize these changes. They orient us to the new landscape, and they point the way through the difficult terrain ahead. As we set out, we become agents in our own lives, not just passive receptacles for grief, but people who *grieve*. As such, it was much easier for me to grieve for my father than it was to grieve for James. How do you even *start* to go about grieving for someone who never lived outside the womb? Who do you call?

In February of 2001, my wife Lisa was in the twentieth week of her first pregnancy when the ultrasound showed no movement and no fetal heartbeat. Offered the choice between a D & C and inducing labor, I assumed we would opt for the surgical procedure. *Why*, I thought, *should Lisa go through the pain of childbirth*? But Lisa, who had carried James, had felt her body change in order to bear him, and had felt him quicken—a featherlight touch—was determined to give birth to him. She wanted to see him. More than that, she felt an urgent need to protect him from harm.

We went home, put together an overnight bag, returned to the hospital, and checked into the maternity wing—the same routine you would follow if you were expecting to bear a living child. Lisa and I were surrounded by some of the same nurses and midwives who would see us through our second child's birth a year later. They gave us a private room and put a marker on the door, a drawing of a teddy bear with a blue ribbon, to alert doctors and technicians that, in this room, things were different. They formed a kind of protective cordon around us, giving what comfort they could and seeing Lisa through what proved to be a relatively short but intensely painful labor. Still, all night, through the walls came the muffled sounds of other women in various stages of labor and, now and then, the distant cry of a newborn.

The next morning, James was born. Gently unfolding his limbs, the midwife laid out his body on a small white towel. She explained to us that he was anencephalic, that he had died, probably about a week earlier, because his nervous system had failed to develop. She handed him to me. Though the mask of his face was perfectly composed, I could see that the back of his head had not fully formed. Serene, thin, nearly translucent, he was perfect. Proportioned less like a baby than a scale model of an older child, he was about the length of my hand. His toes were like mine, the second toe longer than the first.

The midwife left us alone so that we could say good-bye to him. Not knowing what else to do, I passed him to Lisa. She held him, not as she would have held a baby in her arms—he was too small and delicate for that—but as she might have cradled an injured sparrow in her palm. After all that she had been through to see him, I thought Lisa would spend more time with James, but after only a minute or two she asked me to call for the midwife. Later,

Lisa told me he looked so fragile that she was afraid he would come apart in her hand. Carefully handing his body back to the midwife, Lisa asked her to promise to look after him, to see that he was treated with respect.

The hospital released James's body to the funeral home, and a few days later, we went there to arrange for his cremation. The young man who helped us seemed just out of college. Wearing a cheap tie and an ill-fitting suit, it was clear that he hadn't had much experience. Thinking perhaps that he could somehow normalize the situation, he tried to draw us into pleasant conversation. I nodded and said a few things in return, trying to put him at his ease, but Lisa just stared at him. Even under the best of circumstances, my wife does not suffer fools gladly, and it was plain that she wanted to kill him. Still chattering nervously, he showed us into a room that clearly had been designed for large groups, extended families, to gather and plan elaborate services. Seating us at the enormous conference table, he offered us coffee. I declined politely as Lisa sobbed. After a moment, I suggested he should probably just get us the forms to sign.

He excused himself, and we sat quietly for a while, just the two of us, staring at the vast expanse of table before us. Off to our left, a display case featured a selection of urns. Religious urns, urns for two, marble urns, shiny metal urns, biodegradable urns. One had a motorized revolving top with a little landscape: boulders, a gnarled tree, and a bald eagle with wings outstretched. The motor made a little whirring sound, and with each revolution, the urn emitted a series of tiny squeaks, as if the mechanism were in need of a spot of WD-40. We burst out laughing.

We had not quite contained ourselves by the time the young man returned with the forms. He stopped short in the doorway, as if he had somehow blundered into the wrong room. I waved him in, and, my shoulders still shaking, I signed the form authorizing James's cremation on the blank labeled "father." It was the first time anyone had referred to me as a father, and I wondered whether it would be the last.

For the first week after James's birth, Lisa and I stayed home together; we could hardly bear to talk to anyone but each other. Of course, we had to let people at work know we weren't coming in. Lisa teaches yoga, and I am a professor at Saint Martin's, a small Benedictine university south of Seattle. We called our respective bosses, explained the circumstances, and asked them to let our students know that we would be back as soon as possible. We told our parents and a few close friends, but apart from that inner circle, hardly anyone had known that Lisa had been pregnant in the first place. This created an insurmountable, absurd difficulty—a "good news/bad news" story so wild that we couldn't bear to tell it to anyone else.

We hadn't kept the pregnancy a secret exactly, not after the first trimester. Perhaps the reason we hadn't told more people was that it had been so difficult for us to conceive. With the monthly cycle of hope and disappointment and the increasing medicalization of the process over the years, our struggle to conceive became intensely private, and so our success was private as well.

And now, so was our grief. The nurses at the hospital had referred us to counselors and social workers. They gave us a list of books to read and websites to visit. It's not that there aren't resources available to people who have had similar experiences. Whatever your ache, loss, or unfulfilled desire may be, you'll find people out there on the Web who have banded together. Need someone to talk to? There are meetings to attend, phone numbers to call.

We availed ourselves of none of these resources. It just did not occur to us to do so, any more than it would occur to a man who has just been struck by lightning to drag himself, clothes still smoking, to a support group. We sat very still on the couch, the clock ticking on the mantelpiece. Sleep was a relief. To be awake was to look inward, constantly trying to assess the damage.

The following Monday, I went back to work. Lisa remained home. It wasn't only that she needed time to physically recover. She just wasn't ready to be out in a world where people were moving about as if nothing had happened. Though I had a similar dread of facing the workaday world, I was more frightened by my own immobility. Ready or not, I wanted to be back on my feet.

At work, I taught my first class of the day without incident, but soon afterward I found myself in my office, the door closed, staring blankly at the backlog of e-mail on my computer screen. I realized I couldn't carry on the pretense that nothing had happened, but neither could I face going from office to office and dropping the dead weight of the story on each of my friends and coworkers in turn.

I had to let people know somehow, so I composed an e-mail saying simply that our son, James, had been stillborn last week and asking people to hold us in their hearts. I intended to send it only to the people I had told about the pregnancy, but then I couldn't remember which people I had told and which I hadn't. Sitting paralyzed, my hands motionless on the keyboard, I grew more and more frustrated. Finally, I clicked on the e-mail program's address book and sent the message to everyone at the university: faculty, staff, students, people I knew, people I had never met, everyone.

Some people were offended, I know. No one told me so directly, but my department's administrative assistant said later that she received a few e-mails asking who the hell I was. And I'm sure there were many others who felt it was inappropriate to broadcast such personal news via mass e-mail. I thought it was inappropriate too, but given that the only alternative seemed to be silence, I was too angry to care.

For weeks afterward, nearly every day, people at work—some of whom I barely knew—would approach me in the hall or come into my office, softly shutting the door behind them, and burst into tears. And out would spill the stories of their own lost children: miscarriages, babies lost in the second trimester, babies brought to full term. Some of the losses were recent, some years gone by. And they all said the hardest thing was telling people. You haul around this grief, all the time, and there's no place to put it, no one to help you set it down.

I suppose everyone grieves in different ways and at different rates. I threw myself into work, Lisa into solitude. We retrieved James's ashes, about a teaspoonful, from the funeral home. To keep him close, Lisa put the small box in the drawer of her nightstand. When she was well enough, Lisa worked in the garden, planting, weeding, hauling around stones and soil in the freezing March drizzle. At first, she envisioned a memorial garden for James, but the garden felt too big and too far away for such a small soul.

I found some solace, some measure of completion, in hearing others' stories, but I don't know that Lisa's grieving was ever completed so much as it was overruled. In May she got pregnant with Benjamin, and, as she had been with James, she was unremittingly ill for the entire first trimester and beyond. Then, at 26 weeks, part of the placenta suddenly detached from the uterine wall. A rush of blood; the ambulance ride to the hospital; the operating room with the doctors prepped to perform an emergency C-section. The nurse helped me into a set of surgical scrubs. Fortunately, they didn't need to operate; they stopped the bleeding in time. But Lisa spent the next ten weeks in the hospital, strapped to a fetal heart monitor, on constant alert for any sign of distress.

Through it all, Ben was fine, has always been fine. In this story, as in so many of our stories these days, he is the happy ending. Once Benjamin was born, the plans for James's memorial garden were put aside; at once, that patch of real estate had other purposes: strawberry plants, a sandbox, a fort with a trapdoor. We hadn't forgotten James's death, but such a sudden abundance of life made us move on.

It was six years before it occurred to me to write about James. I was teaching a writing class in collaboration with two colleagues from the English department, and we had agreed that we would do each others' writing assignments. I showed a draft of my homework to Lisa in order to check my facts, and she remarked that I ought to try to get it published. The essay languished on my hard drive for more than a year before, on a whim, I submitted it. And that was how Lisa and I went from telling no one what had happened to telling the entire readership of the Sunday *New York Times*.[1]

The first e-mail came from Australia, where Sunday arrives nineteen hours sooner than it does in Seattle. For weeks afterward, people sent me their stories, literally from all over the world. Some had lost a child as recently as the week before. One man was mourning a stillbirth that had happened sixty years ago. He had never wept about it until he read the *Times* article, and he'd never discussed it with anyone, not even his wife—and now she was gone. He'd always thought that none of his friends or family had been through a similar experience, but now he had to wonder.

Though no one contacted me directly to say so, the article offended some people. One man wrote to the *Times*, taking me to task for misspelling *anencephalic* (I had spelled it "anacephalic," which is indeed incorrect); he suggested that, had I truly cared about the welfare of my son, I would have taken the trouble to learn the spelling of the condition that killed him. I considered writing back and, in the most civil terms, asking for his forgiveness for the error; I had gotten the spelling off my son's death certificate.

The blogosphere was similarly bizarre. Once the article had been posted on the *Times* website, it was reposted on a number of sites where readers were invited to post comments. For the most part, people responded as you might expect: with sadness and with their own stories of stillbirth and other losses. However, one post suggested that Lisa and I were foolish to go through the birth process, that we had taken unnecessary risks with her health (untrue), and that we were in love with death. In each string of comments, it seemed, there was at least one anonymous post so heartless and wrathful that it would make any sane reader want to give his fellow citizens a wide berth.

As I had referred to James as a child, not a fetus, inevitably some of the repostings were in service of pro-life groups, and the article was cited in various antiabortion screeds. Even though we had expected this to happen, Lisa and I found this particular extrapolation from the personal to the political both intrusive and offensive—a kind of kidnapping. Believe what you like, say what you want, but leave my son out of it.

Not long ago, I got an e-mail from a woman asking me how Lisa and I respond when people ask us how many children we have. I replied that, given that the question is usually asked in the context of small talk, we just say "One"—Benjamin. We're no longer mourning James, and it doesn't feel right to us to drop his death into casual conversation. Not in this society, not in this age, so violent and yet so detached from the quotidian reality of death, so unversed in grieving. Telling the simple truth becomes an assault.

It wasn't always so. Would that, when asked about her children, a woman were still able to say, as women used to say, simply: "I have seven, four living."

CHAPTER FOUR

The Traumatic Contradiction: When Birth and Death Collide

Joanne Cacciatore

> Probably there is nothing in human nature more resonant with charges than the flow of energy between two biologically alike bodies, one of which has lain in amniotic bliss inside the other, one of which has laboured to give birth to the other. The materials are here for the deepest mutuality and the most painful estrangement.
>
> —Adrienne Rich, feminist and author

The Colliding

The day of birth is a zenith, often celebrated, revered, and ritualized across cultures throughout history. But for some women, an unwelcome intruder imposes Himself in that liminal space between death and birth, and there the two great mysteries, commingled, become one.

I found out I was pregnant on Thanksgiving Day 1993. It was an uneventful pregnancy filled with the usual distractions of a young, thriving, and adventurous family. So every month, as if a new family ritual, I gathered my three young children for prenatal appointments. They were enthralled with my expanding belly, giggling as they imagined the baby dancing inside me. We regularly listened with a Doppler to her beating heart. We shared our dreams and hopes for the newest member of our family. And with only two weeks to go, the three children, aged three, five, and six, lovingly helped decorate the nursery, with neutral tones of dancing bears and pastel balloons. The final weeks were filled with the repetitive inquiries of three very anxious children, as if on a prolonged road trip to an exciting destination, "Mommy, when will the baby be here? When will the baby be here?!"

On July 27, 1994, the due date of my baby, I went to the hospital, car seat loaded and bags packed, pains coming more frequently than they should for such a long drive. I arrived and was immediately taken to labor and delivery. The pain of the transitional contractions was agonizing, the waves coming furiously one after the other. And then, though the memories of the event fade in and out of the shadows of my mind, I vaguely remember hearing the words that would forever change my life: "We can't find the baby's heartbeat." Surely, there must be some mistake. *These people are crazy*, I thought to myself, trying to focus on breathing through each unrelenting contraction. Sweat rolled down my face—pushing, pushing, pushing, and within minutes, she emerged from my Judas body. "Breathe, baby, breathe," I whispered to myself. I waited to hear something, anything. The silence was heavy, pressing down on my chest. With my eyes closed, my fists clenched, and legs shaking uncontrollably, I was paralyzed with fear, waiting to hear the familiar cries of a newborn baby. Still, silence, deafening silence, for what seemed like hours. Terror descended over me, and I felt myself leave my body.

A voice cracked the silence, like a rock shattering glass: "Your baby is dead. Do you want to see the baby?" *What?* I thought to myself, *What are they saying? Why are they lying to me?*

I tried to get up from the bed and leave. I wanted to go home. My baby could not be dead. This could not be happening to me. *If only I could leave, go home to bed, and wake up tomorrow,* I thought to myself, *it would all be OK.*

Someone, I don't remember who because their faces were blurs of unfamiliar flesh, wrapped the baby, all eight pounds and twenty-two inches of her, in a blanket. "You have a beautiful baby girl," said the faceless voice, and I sat up and opened my eyes. I reached my disbelieving arms to embrace the lifeless body of my daughter. My forty long weeks of tireless work had come to an end without my due reward. As I took her in my arms, I was overcome with both pride and sorrow. She was the most beautiful baby I'd ever seen. Her name, Cheyenne, means "mourning dove."

I didn't sleep for three days following her birth and death. I couldn't eat or listen to music. Everything hurt. Even breathing hurt, and in my anguish, I scribbled these words:

Thirty-Three Hours

It is 3:04 a.m.
Only 33 hours since your birth . . .

And your death.
But it seems an eternity.

Still I hope to awaken from this nightmare
To find myself pregnant
And complaining about your knee in my rib, again.

I have always known
That losing a child
Would be the most difficult experience for a parent to endure.
Yet I never imagined the pain would feel so much like terror.

So I live and relive the hours before your birth and death
Wondering,
Was it something I ate?
Or lifted or said?
Desperately clinging to theories on
Why you couldn't hold onto life.

I only know that from the moment of your miraculous existence
Inside of me,
I loved you intensely.

Just as the other three whom I so deeply love
I also loved and needed you.

And each day I dreamed and planned for your future.
Your kindergarten class
Graduation
College
Your wedding day.
Even your own children. But I never planned for your death.
Now, I ache for you
Beautiful Cheyenne.
My arms long desperately to hold you and to love you.

I long to kiss your soft skin and stroke your cheek as I nurse you at my breast.
I long to rock you to sleep and sing you the "raindrops on roses" song
(It is your big sister's favorite)

I long to see you growing every day,
Playing with your sister and brothers,
Filling our days with your laughter and our nights with your love.

I long to take you on walks to the park.
and see the glimmering sun in your beautiful eyes.

I long to awaken you every morning
With a smile and a kiss (or two)

But your death has left me with an empty womb and a broken heart.
Wondering if the sun will ever shine again
Or if the sparrow's song will ever sound as sweet.

Wondering if each and every smile will always be this painful
And each tear as heart wrenching.

And though others may,
I will not forget you, little girl.
Nor do I wish to try.

I will love you and keep you
Close to my heart
Until my last
Dying breath . . .

Forever Yours,
Mommy

One week later, on a sweltering summer day, I buried my little girl in a pink satin casket, as my breasts, engorged with her milk, burned in protest. My arms ached, my chest felt hollow, and I could barely speak. I lay sobbing on her grave, amidst the smell of freshly cut grass, as my tears consorted with the dirt, and begged the God in whom I hadn't believed to give her back. I was among the living dead, reminded of what Saint Francis meant when he said that once you've faced the Great Death, the second death is of no consequence. I was estranged from myself, catapulted into an epic existential crisis that would change the course of my life. Yes, I knew that I would never again be the same person.

Three weeks after her death, I received a document from the Arizona Office of Vital Records. I thought it was her birth certificate, the only document I would have to place in her baby book, an emotional artifact evidencing her existence. To my dismay, it was, instead, a death certificate. I called to inquire and was told that I would not get a certificate of birth since I "didn't really have a baby." Further investigations confirmed this fact. No state in the United States allowed women to request and pay for a certificate of birth for a stillborn baby. My daughter had been reduced to an asterisk, not worthy of any type of dignified recognition. I was plagued with platitudes, from the delivery man to the grocery clerk to family members: "God has a plan for you," or "Everything happens for a reason," or "You're young and can have more," and even "God needed an angel to tend His garden." None of it made sense, and I began to withdraw from situations in which I'd encounter others.

The incessant questions I asked myself about why she died as well as the loneliness of my very private grief overcame me. Within a month after her death, my weight had dropped dangerously low and I wasn't certain if I was going to survive. One very late night in September of 1994, while grieving in the dark corner on the floor of my closet, I made a promise to her that if I survived, when I was stronger, I would help others. I vowed that her life would have meaning because she did, in fact, exist. And I embarked on the most painfully beautiful journey I could have ever imagined.

In 1996, while I was pregnant with her baby brother, Cheyenne's death gave birth to the MISS Foundation, an international organization for bereaved families that offers counseling, advocacy, research, and education (C.A.R.E.) after the death of a child at any age and from any cause. The organization has grown quickly to seventy-four chapters around the world, with twenty-seven online support groups and a website that receives more than one million visitors a month. I didn't name the organization after her. I didn't need for her name to be known or for others to focus on her. For me, it wasn't about that. I just needed to know, quietly within my heart, that she mattered, and that in her mattering she could touch the world in some small way through service to others who were suffering.

The Explosion

One of the unique features of losing a child to stillbirth is the lack of societal understanding around this type of traumatic death. It is often minimized, hushed into the taxonomy of pregnancy loss, rather than what it *really* is—the death of a baby. This collision of birth and death is not something uttered in childbirth education classes or at the local mom support group, so many women don't even realize, despite the data, that stillbirth still occurs with relative frequency in contemporary society. And in so many ways, women who experience stillbirth are invalidated, under-researched, and disenfranchised.

Stillbirth has always been the "dirty family secret" about which no one would speak; this attitude shamed women into quietly mourning their losses with the same silence in which their dead children were born.

But the face of stillbirth is rapidly changing. The twenty-first century has brought a modern-day maternal revolution as women who have experienced stillbirth struggle for respect and validation. These changes are giving women the lexica—psychologically sophisticated language—to speak about their losses. And when we can find words to capture an experience, society's responses to those experiences often begin to evolve toward a framework of understanding and respect.

Part of this respect gained momentum in Arizona in 1999 when I began lobbying to change the law regarding the way stillbirths are recorded by the state. I marshaled a coalition to address the long-standing policies precluding the issuance of a birth certificate for stillborn infants. The team was made up of a pediatrician, a neonatologist, a medical examiner, an attorney, a social worker, and seven women who had experienced stillbirth. We assessed potential roadblocks and identified stakeholders for the next six months, then strategized. I went to work garnering supporters for the legislation that was soon to become House Bill 2416—the MISSing Angels Bill. We were completely unaware of the widespread reform we were about to incite. HB2416 would allow women and their partners to request and pay for a Certificate of Birth Resulting in Stillbirth (CBRS) after the stillbirth of a baby.

We contended that the passage of HB2416 would encourage more standardized data collection statewide. The CBRS would collect more maternal and familial health data, which might then lead to research opportunities and an enhanced understanding of the causes and trends in stillbirth and diagnoses of death. And there are psychological benefits to the issuance of the CBRS. The policies mandating (1) economic responsibility of final disposition and (2) the issuance of a death certificate, absent acknowledgment of the birth, were no longer acceptable to many women. One mother said of her experience:

> The fact that the state simply offered me a death certificate, a constant reminder of my failure, caused me great emotional pain. This bill was important to me for many reasons, not the least of which is that this legislation recognizes a traditionally illegitimate loss, and resultant grief, for me and for thousands of women. It acknowledges a very significant event—birth. A mother of a stillborn must still give birth to her dead infant.
>
> —Heidi, Phoenix, Arizona

Finally, the CBRS is the only logical political course to follow. Interestingly, a premature infant weighing less than one pound and born at 19 weeks' gestation, who takes one laborious breath yet has no chance at survival outside the womb, will receive a Certificate of Live Birth. Conversely, a baby born at 42 weeks' gestation who dies just one minute prior to birth and weighs ten pounds would receive only a certificate of fetal death.

So in June of 2001, after we spent more than a year educating legislators about the trauma of stillbirth, Governor Jane D. Hull signed HB2416, the MISSing Angels Bill, into law. As she signed the document, Hull said, "I think we all know that this change is something that should have happened a long time ago." Since its inception and enactment, twenty-four other states (including Massachusetts, California, and New Jersey) have passed similar legislation. In most states, little or no opposition came from concerned stakeholders. We would go on to pass other legislation related to stillbirth in Arizona. In 2002, we passed SB2001, the Sudden Infant Death Advisory Council, whose expanded charge was to investigate deaths of babies from stillbirth to age three. The committee would extrapolate data and report findings to the governor in an effort to reduce the number of sudden infant deaths in Arizona. In May of 2004, Governor Janet Napolitano signed SB1003 into law, an act that would allow for a one-time tax deduction of $2,300 for families experiencing stillbirth during the same year in which the birth and death occurred. And for the first time in history, Dr. Duane Alexander, director of the National Institutes of Health (NIH), responding to the outcry of thousands of stillbirth women and their families, announced that his agency had included stillbirth in its research agenda for the fiscal year 2002. This trend has continued into the most recent NIH budget.

Yes, the movement toward broader, long-awaited recognition of stillborn babies and their mothers is well on its way. Today, I am a tenure-track professor, researcher, and death studies educator at Arizona State University. In the past several years, I've published seven articles specifically about perinatal death in peer-reviewed journals. Other researchers around the country are becoming increasingly interested in this taboo subject and its survivors, and eventually, the once-hidden tragedy of stillbirth that was so misunderstood will be saliently present in the literature, worthy of the same dignity and recognition as any other child's life and death. And I spend many days counseling mothers and fathers whose babies and children have died. While there is much work to be done, I am hopeful that, at last, the shroud of silence around stillbirth has been lifted.

The Orbit

There are some losses, some grief experiences, so profoundly painful, that there simply are no words to describe it, no sounds to express it, and for many, no God who can heal it. No magical pill can vanquish it. I buried her on August 1, 1994, surrendering her thirty-two-inch-long pink satin coffin to the men in gray suits. They lowered her casket into the ground, and I felt myself lunge toward her, like elastic returning to its natural state. Every cell in my body was programmed to be *with* her.

Death trespassed on my body. Just moments before I was to bring forth life, Death came into my body and without permission stole my most precious piece of my self. My beautiful girl, all eight pounds, with long, piano fingers, ebony curls, and fat creased thighs, succumbed to that which cannot be contained. Still, I can't *really* describe the trauma of experiencing birth in such intimate proximity to death.

It has taken me years to come to terms with all that I lost that July day in 1994, pieces of the ongoing pain imbibed from others. Hurried and unknowing voices told me what I should and shouldn't do, how to mourn and how not to mourn, when to remember and when to forget. They told me it would be bad for my children to see her lifeless body. It would cause them grief beyond repair. How would I know it was the not-seeing that would cause much greater harm? I'd wanted to bring her body home for a day, show her the room that was to hold her cradle. Let her witness all the hours I'd meticulously spent cutting brown bear borders against the cornflower blue walls, until my fingertips blistered. They said I couldn't, I shouldn't, and I didn't. Mostly, I wanted to cremate her and have her at home, close to me, where she belonged. But others thought it would be "bad for me." As often in the early days of grief, my desires were defeated without a fight. After all, battling requires sentience and strength, and I had neither. My emotions were being managed by others, coerced into convivial proscriptions of comfortability. And Death, like a neglectful parent both loved and hated, held the key to both my freedom and my confinement. I felt condemned to a purgatorial space between life and death from which I could not expiate myself.

But gradually through the years I made space for living again. Grief moved aside years ago, and joy stands as a comrade next to *my* grief. My grief—it was mine. I earned it, I owned it. And it eventually became my friend, too. I'm not sure how, but I survived for nearly sixteen years. In the blink of an eye, nearly six thousand days have passed absent the presence of one of my precious children. But not a single second of any hour of any day of any month of any year have I not been cognizant of her absence. As C. S. Lewis said, "Her absence is like the sky, spread over everything." And I've tried to make good on the promises I made her in 1994 while I sat on my closet floor.

One of those promises came to fruition in April of 2008. I had Cheyenne disinterred. Her pink coffin was freed from the ground, and I brought her back from the men in gray suits. And for one week, I had the chance to experience my own trauma and regrief on my own terms. It was much more difficult than I could have imagined it would be, the innards of my grief raw and exposed again to the light. But it was *my* way, with no one telling me I couldn't rock her in unison with the neighbor's cottonwood tree that swung in the wind. No one telling me that a one-way conversation with my dead child's own lovely bones would be plain crazy. No one telling me that I should scurry my children out the door, protect them from the pains of loving, shelter them from grief. I held power over my experiences this time, mindfully experiencing it in full.

I was able to burn my sage and follow my mind down the rabbit hole. I took my time, fell asleep with my hand on the pink satin box, where I'd earlier tied purple bows in knots to abate the morbid inquisitions of others, and myself. And I captured my first photograph of all five children gathered together, four of whom emerged from my womb safely and one who would never smell the blossoming jasmine, hear the coyotes howling behind our home, or taste the crunchy bittersweetness of a ripened pomegranate. In some small way, I feel like now she's closer to where she's belonged all these years. She's come full circle: home. And for this, I am grateful. Her cremains are now always close, down the stairs, around the corner, in her 125-year-old cherrywood butsudan.

The beauty is finally bigger than the pain . . .

The Ascension

My mothering of Cheyenne did not end on that hot summer day in July of 1994. Sixteen years later, I continue to discover new meanings and insights about our unique relationship. I am continually receiving what I call her gifts. She has taught me more in her brief time on earth than I could have taught her in a lifetime: that love is unconditional, that you cannot sit back and watch injustice, that death is not to be feared, that it is OK to dance in the rain, that time is merely perception, that one person can truly change the world, that kindnesses last forever, that words *can* break bones, and that the wounded need others.

Euphemisms don't ease the suffering of the bereaved. Telling someone that "God has a plan," or that "They're in a better place," is not helpful to many grieving people. It is simply a way to avoid painful but honest conversations about mortality, loss, and suffering. The best thing we can do for the bereaved is to offer unconditional support; to leave our hearts open to them and our ears ready to listen with a fully compassionate presence; and of course, to recognize both the value of the relationship that has been lost and grief as a normal response to that loss.

My love for her did not end with her death, as the sun does not end with its setting. It is much, much bigger than that. It is never-ending, enduring, faithful. One day in the future, when I'm an old woman, perhaps only moments from my final breath, someone will ask me about my life on earth and I will say, as I always have, without wavering, "I have five children."

And I will have loved her and kept her close to my heart until my last dying breath . . . just as I promised.

CHAPTER FIVE

Living with (and without) Caleb

Kelley Krahling

I suppose in a perfect world, I could write a story with a beginning, a middle, and an end. But I do not live in a perfect world. You do not live in a perfect world. We do not live in a perfect world. And as I have come to learn, very few stories—true stories, that is—come in perfect packages, neatly told and tidily finished. Stories live. They evolve. And they never end.

The real story of my Caleb doesn't have words and it continues on each day, even though he is long gone from me—physically gone, that is. I guess that is what becomes so hard. As each day passes he slips farther away from my physical self. The memory of his kicks and rolls within me dims and is overshadowed by the nightmare of his birth. The moment of feeling him literally slip out of my body and away from this earth. The hollowness of my empty belly, the numbness of my legs and mind—this is what I remember.

The hospital room was quiet. It was only my husband, the nurse, and me. When my first two babies, my son and my daughter, were born, our whole family was there, waiting. A waiting room full of grandparents, aunts, uncles, and as the years passed, big brothers and sisters, all ready to welcome a new life. But not this time. Not for Caleb.

I found out at a routine doctor's appointment that he had died; I walked into the appointment expressing concerns that my baby had not been moving as much as usual. The ultrasound technician dismissed my worries easily, barely even giving them notice. And then, mere minutes later, she grabbed my hand and asked beseechingly, "If the news is bad, is there anyone here with you?" And then I was abandoned in the exam room, my still pregnant and full belly exposed, the silent ultrasound machine next to me, and all I could think was "FUCK!" And almost simultaneously the thought "How am I going to tell my kids?" spun inside my head.

I called my husband and no one else; he told everyone else. I felt the need to hide myself and my son away from the world. All I knew was that in those moments, in those hours after I had been told that my baby had died, I wanted to be away, far, far away from everywhere, from everyone. I was scared, I was weak, and I was alone. A room full of people could not have made me feel less alone than I felt in those hours. I was the wounded animal who cowers, seeking a secluded shelter from the world. I wanted to be tucked away in a dark box under the stove, left to die or live, without intervention. I didn't want it to feel better, ever.

I closed my eyes. I literally pulled the covers over my eyes. I gave birth to Caleb in the early morning hours of Labor Day, September 1, 2007. The story of his birth isn't chronicled in a bound baby book or recorded on video to replay on his birthday. He was born into an obnoxiously bright room, despite the curtains being drawn against the insistent late summer sun. It was quiet. Our nurse, who had been with us through a long night's labor, checked me and told me that it was time to push. My husband, who had finally succumbed to sleep just a short while before, was across the room from me, uncomfortably curled on the couch. I cried out for him. He came to me and folded me into his chest. The nurse told me to push when I was ready. I would never be ready. Ever. But my body defied my heart, defied my will, defied my mind.

And he was born.

The announcement by our nurse of his previously unknown gender wasn't one made in exclamation or congratulations. We received the news only because I asked her, "Is it a boy?" I had known all along that he was, indeed, a boy. She nodded in affirmation as she wrapped his tiny body in a blanket and asked me, "Did you know?" I told her I did, but not because of any test or scan but because I knew, in my heart, that he was a boy. I knew. I always knew. I don't know how long we spent in that room with him. That room that had felt so gross and dark to me when I walked into it hours before (literally becoming ill at the sight of a room that had before brought two healthy, living children into my life and would soon become a place where I gave birth to death, my child's death) had become a place of refuge for me. The room wasn't so scary anymore. It now held me and my child. And as much as I wanted it to be dark, there it was, the light, an unwelcome guest in my life, and it surrounded us. There it was. Dawn. And birth. Still. Birth.

He was my son. I needed to love him. I needed to be with him. I needed to be his mother. I lay on the bed with him next to me; I looked at him and tried to memorize everything about him. I remember thinking how much he looked like his sister. His nose, his mouth: hers in miniature. I knew two things. He was perfect. And he was dead. And after some amount of time, I have no idea how much, the nurse asked us if we were ready to say good-bye or if we wanted to spend more time with him. And somehow—to this day I don't know how—we said we were ready to leave him. He was taken away from us and I was cleaned up. The nurses and other hospital staff moved me to a gurney. My legs were still paralyzed from the epidural. As they opened the door to our room that September morning and started to wheel me out to relocate me to a more "appropriate" wing of the hospital (one where I wouldn't be surrounded by healthy, screaming new babies and tired but blissfully ignorant new mothers), in a sad and desperate attempt to shield myself from the world, I pulled the thin hospital sheet over my head and I closed my eyes.

In the beginning, recovering didn't even seem like an option. It is a concept that you can't even grasp. In the beginning, you want the darkness to swallow you whole and never spit you out. But as the long, hard days and even darker, endless nights stretch out and become weeks and then months, you find yourself struggling to be free of the darkness once more. Is the daylight more appealing? Not really, but the cold, shadowy pit of grief has become less comforting, and so you seek an alternate place of refuge. And you rejoin the world of the living because it is no longer the people you want to hide from but your feelings. All of them.

Those first few weeks of surviving between the night and the day, the dark and the light, were for me the most trying and exhausting days of my life. After the immediacy of the days surrounding losing Caleb were over, the days when I buried my head and my heart, my former life beckoned me. My children cried out for me. I went to them. And it took every ounce of energy I had to get up each day and function, even at the barest minimum. To talk with other parents, to drive, to attend meetings and sporting events, to plan, to execute, to grocery shop, to make any decisions at all, sucked what little life I had within me right back out. It wasn't until December, almost four months after Caleb's birth, that I stopped moving long enough to let myself breathe. And then I collapsed, physically and mentally.

Autopilot shut off and I went down. I needed to. Christmas morning, after all the presents were opened and everyone was happily engaged with all things new, I climbed back into my bed, closed my eyes, and imagined myself far, far away from all of it, from all of them. I closed my eyes and pretended that none of them existed. I was away from everything I knew and loved and it was just me. In my mind, for those moments, I walked alone. I was the me I used to be, before I said, "I do," before I said, "We're having a baby!" Before.

. . . I fancied all sorts of crazy futures for myself. I tried to imagine my life without everything that was my life.

And then I slept. I slept for days. I got up only to do what had to be done. And then I slept some more. I didn't stay that way for long, but it was long enough to remind me that there is a lot more to healing than just waking up every day.

And there still is more. There will always be more.

I think from the outside to the casual and even not-so-casual observer, I appear healed.

I'm not.

But I am not anywhere near the same place I was that day he was born. My life has evolved, moved on, continued. Really, when you think about it, there were only two choices: find a way to go forward, or die. I chose the former. I *had* to. I had two other children who needed me to. I don't know, honestly, what I would have done if they hadn't needed me. I don't know how far I would have fallen, how deep the depression would have taken me. Since losing Caleb, I have come to know and befriend other mothers who have lost their first babies and have somehow found their way out of hell. I like to imagine that I would have, too, had Caleb been my first. But none of us ever really knows how we would carry someone else's burden. We know our own life—we take what is thrown at us and we try to figure out how to muddle through. We stumble, we falter, we collapse. And then, somehow, we get up. Maybe it's a hand reaching through the darkness, or a voice calling out to us that reminds us we aren't alone. Maybe it's sheer force of will. Or a combination of all of it. The knowing that there are others out there, the desire to start anew, the absolute determination not to give up. At least not yet.

And it is all of that—all of that hard work; the inner battle of demons; the taking on of forces beyond our control; the daily, sometimes hourly or even the minute-by-minute, second-by-second fight to survive, to continue, to exist—it is all of that, that people don't see. It is that entire emotional rebuilding, piece by tiny piece that they don't get, that they can never understand. And it is in missing this part of the journey that makes it so easy for people to caricature a baby-loss mom as some sort of misfit, a character in an episodic tragedy. "Oh, her baby died, that's why she is __________." It makes for a convenient story line, a wonderful tragic event that turns the best, most capable woman into a weeping pile of compost, no longer able to function in a "normal" world.

After Caleb's birth, I watched the season finale of ABC's *Private Practice*. One of the main characters, a psychiatrist, is pregnant, and one of her patients shows up at the psychiatrist's house with a needle full of drugs. She intends to literally rip the baby out of the main character's belly. Why? Because the patient's baby had died and, obviously, that is what moms of babies who have died do. We wander the earth seeking out other pregnant moms who must be carrying our babies and then we slice them open and take what is rightfully ours.

It's a cheap shot. It's easy. And, yes, I suppose it sells. But it's not real. And it humiliates all of us; it humiliates every mother who has somehow navigated the shitstorm of losing a child, of giving birth to a dead baby, and has—step by painstaking, fucking step—regained a life. It is not the story we wanted, it is not the life story we planned, but still, it is our life. And we aren't a bunch of demented, crazy mothers who wander around, crazily hunting down pregnant women in a deluded effort to reclaim our dead babies. We deserve better than this. So much better than this story told about us.

My life since Caleb has been a mighty struggle. This isn't to say that it hasn't gotten easier—because it has. I am no longer consumed by his death. His death no longer stops me from living my life. Nor does it stop me from believing that I can have a life. A good life, a great life, even. But nonetheless, it is a struggle. Thoughts of him, memories of the day he was born—they hover around my head like a song quietly playing in the background. Sometimes I can tune it out, and other times I can't. But, some days, most days, are infinitely better than others.

It has taken a lot for me to get here. It has been—and continues to be—a process. Getting here, living my life as a mother of a stillborn baby, is still happening. I didn't get here by accident or by design but I did get here. Where is *here*? It is ordinary. It is day-to-day. It is nothing special and yet it is still extraordinary. It's not locked up in a padded room, it is not seeking out the pregnant woman who has somehow stolen my baby and tucked it away into her uterus. It is not a vengeful, unfeeling, demented woman. I wish people could see that far from the extremes of batshit-crazy there exists the lot of us, the moms of dead babies who quietly wander the world. And I wish that they could see us for who we really are.

I wish there were a way to explain what living with the loss of your child is like. I wish that, every once in a while, the world would stop. I wish that, in that moment, I could show you what it is that I, that we, have lived through. I wish that I could show you all that I lost, and I wish that I could show you, that I could introduce you to, the child that I am living without. I wish. I wish . . .

There is no real healing when you lose a child. There is no point in time when you are able to evaluate your loss and make peace with it. At least, not for me. It will never be OK; it will never sit comfortably in my cache of emotional baggage as something I have gotten over. Yes, I have resumed my life; I have laughed again, I have been silly, I have thrown a party or two, and I have even had another baby—but none of those things has made any difference in the loss of my son Caleb. His absence is still enormous. I look at my three living children as they play together, the two older ones fawning over their little brother, and I see him, I see Caleb, not there. I even stop myself sometimes when I think how happy it makes me to see them all together and I think of him, not here, missing the tickles of his siblings, missing their light kisses on his head, missing their continuous antics to make a giggle erupt, and I think how robbed he was, how robbed we all were. My oldest child, my first son, who never talks about Caleb unless prompted, recently said to me out of nowhere, "I wish we had them both here, Mom," and I knew that it is not just me who feels Caleb's absence.

A day has not gone by that I haven't thought of him, missed him, and yearned for him. I think people believe that losing a baby, a child, is like any other death. They acknowledge the greater tragedy, but not the greater grief. There is more to baby loss, child loss, than the loss. There is the living with the loss. The loss kills you. And then somehow, you are resurrected. You find yourself within the shell of who you used to know, all things around you seemingly unchanged; life has gone on and you are standing in the middle of it, stripped bare and empty while still the world requires you to be you. Allotted the "appropriate" grieving time, you then have to get on with it, move on—live, goddamn it, live. And begrudgingly, most of us do. But it takes so much work. Each day we rise and face the sun and we live with it. People have said to me, "I don't know how you do it. I never could have recovered from a loss like that." And I think to myself, *Yes, you would have.* You do somehow recover. You aren't the same person you once were but you find a way, you do find a way to live with it and the person you have become. It doesn't happen overnight, and it doesn't happen just because you want it to.

What makes the grief so hard for me is that there isn't that point to which I can look back and reminisce, no time when I can share fond memories of Caleb and his life. There is no past with which I can comfort myself in the future. His past *is* his death. His tiny, short life within me was just exactly that: within me. No one else shared it. No one else even saw him, only my husband and me. And his pictures are not ones that bring me comfort. Instead, they break me. They reflect a baby who had his life stolen away from him. A perfectly tiny baby with every tiny piece of his body in place, ready to face life—only to have it choked out of him by a cord defect. I can't reminisce or look back fondly on our time together because it all wraps itself in the cloak of Caleb's numbered days with me. With us.

He permeates my being. He is such a huge part of who I am, and yet to most people he doesn't exist. If he is acknowledged at all it is because someone might say or think, "Oh yeah, she is the one whose baby died." That way of remembering Caleb makes it about me and my loss, not about him and what he lost.

I remember sitting with him at the mortuary, holding him, putting the well-worn, favorite, faded, pale blue blanket that was once his big brother's around him, placing the family pictures of all of us by his side. I knew that this was the very last time that I would ever have with him and I wanted to try and tell him how much he was wanted and how much he was, and is, loved. I wanted to tell him everything we ever wanted for him, that we ever dreamed of for him. I wanted to tell him his whole life story; I wanted to give him his lifetime in those moments that we were together. But I had no idea how to do it. And really, there was no way to do it.

My husband, the man who had walked into the dark, still exam room at the doctor's office days earlier and had taken me into his arms; the man who, when I said we have to call my parents, grabbed his cell phone and dialed their number and as the phone at the other end started to ring looked at me and said, "I can't do this, not in front of you," and walked out into the hallway in order to shield me somehow from hearing the news, again, that our child had died; this same man, who made the phone calls to counselors, to mortuaries, to cemeteries, and to so many of our friends, and had to explain *over* and *over* again what had happened, this man drove me to the mortuary, introduced me to someone who had been "handling" our Caleb, then held me as we walked back to a room where our son was, opened the door to the room, walked purposefully to where Caleb lay, bent over and looked at him, and then turned and looked at me and said, "I can't do this." And left.

It was too much. Way too much. So I sat alone with Caleb, just as I sit alone with his memory now, and I tried to make sure that I said the right things, that I told him everything he needed to know and everything I wanted him to hear. I tried to make sure that I did right by him.

Even now as he drifts farther away from me, I feel the need to pull him closer, to make myself remember the tiniest of details about him and his brief time here on this earth. I need to make his life meaningful, to make it matter, to make sure that it is clear he mattered, that he still does and always will matter. I never want anyone to think he is something I got over. I won't. I will live my life without him, every day. And every day I will think of him, I will miss him, I will love him, and I will wish like hell that he were still here. Because I too, want both of them, Caleb and Cason, here.

On September 1, 2007, I gave birth to my son Caleb. He never heard my cries as I felt him leave my body. He never took a breath, cried, or opened his eyes. He never felt my hand as I lifted his foot to look at his tiny perfect toes. He never heard me tell him I love him. But I said it; I said it then and I still do to this day. I whisper it to the winds and to the wide-open skies and hope that he hears it. Hope that he knew, that he still knows.

People say that there isn't a word to describe the pain you feel when you lose a child. In my head I say, *Yes, there is*, and I whisper, "Caleb."

CHAPTER SIX

He Changed Our World

Marion J. Flores

The tundra was thoroughly encased in ice. So frozen, in fact, that the memorial garden where we were burying him needed six days to thaw the ground enough to dig the few feet legally required to bury an infant. My husband, Steve, and I waited in mourning, while the dirt warmed enough from the ground heaters to accept the burial of our first child. He had been stillborn at noon on January 18, 1994, in Madison, Wisconsin, during a deep winter freeze.

With the ground finally dug, nearly thirty members of our family and friends gathered to mourn and support us at Steve II's funeral. Those in attendance gasped as the funeral director instructed me to carry my son's infant-sized, cream-colored casket out of the cemetery's large mausoleum where the service had been held. The crowd waited in silence as I mustered the emotional strength needed to rise from my chair, lift my son's casket, and walk out toward the black Cadillac waiting to transport us to his graveside service. My mother says, "As a mother and grandmother, there is nothing worse than watching your daughter carry a casket containing the child that she grew inside of her. I was aware she had no strength to complete the task, and, as she stumbled repeatedly, I knew there was nothing, absolutely nothing, that could be done to help her pain."

The graveside service was brief, as those in attendance shivered in the below-zero temperatures. The crowd froze in emotional panic as the funeral director instructed me, the grieving mother, to place my child into the ground. Tears poured down as I took the few steps toward the bleak hole that would swallow my son for eternity. I placed my only child's casket into the ground. Wanting to remain with him, I had to be pulled back from the grave by four family members. The subarctic freeze perfectly reflected my emotions during those first months, maybe even years, after the stillbirth of my only biological child.

I delivered him knowing he was not going to survive. The onset of our nightmare had begun four days prior to his birth. I had felt a slight cramping. It was still so early in the pregnancy, I headed to the bathroom. While I was sitting on the toilet, my water broke. As a first-time mother, I was unsure what had occurred. I believed it was simply too early for labor, but I knew something was definitely wrong.

When we arrived at the hospital, we were sent to a perinatology unit. The receptionist advised us that the doctor we were slated to see was in an emergency and we would have to wait. I was extremely uncomfortable and paced the long institutional hallways endlessly because walking relieved my back pain. I was unsure what I was experiencing; I did not realize that it was the contractions of early labor.

When we were finally called into an examination room, a battery of tests was performed. The diagnosis: my cervix was weak and had given way from the weight of the pregnancy. I was given medications to stop the contractions, but we were advised that the little boy growing inside me most likely would not survive without the amniotic fluid. We went home with the knowledge that our son would be delivered extremely prematurely.

I was placed on complete bed rest and advised there was a 90 percent chance my son would be stillborn. As family gathered around us, we prayed nonstop for a miracle. Four days later, I got up to go to the bathroom. While sitting on the toilet I felt something moving between my legs. Terrified, I reached down to feel what was causing the movement; I was too large with pregnancy to look. When I reached down, I felt a tiny foot and toes wiggling between my fingers. My screams summoned my husband and mother. My mother helped me up off the toilet as Steve ran to call 9-1-1.

Critical questions raced through my mind, questions that had never been answered in my many prenatal visits, or in the numerous pregnancy books I had read. Should I keep standing, or could the baby fall out onto the floor? Should I risk sitting down with the baby already descending down the birth canal, or could repositioning break my son's legs, or worse, his neck? What should I do, knowing that he wasn't coming headfirst? Would our son manage to survive, despite the odds?

I stood while my mother knelt in front of me, holding out her hands, in case her grandson started to fall to the floor. Minutes seemed like hours as we waited for the paramedics to make their way through the ice storm that was raging outside. The medical team hovered around me while my son's second leg arrived. They needed to get me to the ambulance, but conditions would not allow use of their stretcher. So they each grabbed one of my limbs and lifted, laying me back as they went. They carried me, naked from the waist down, out of the house and down the pathway, where they shuffled their way across the ice and snow.

Steve and I somberly requested a minister be called to the delivery room. After Steve II's delivery, we were able to hold him and kiss his angelic little face. We held his lifeless body as the minister baptized him. With a nurse's patient guidance we bathed, dressed, and prepared him for his final resting.

We grievingly cherished every moment with him, as our time with him was limited. We were able to collect only a few mementos of his life, proof he ever really existed: his ceremonial birth certificate, baptismal record, death certificate, the shell that held his baptismal water, and a few precious photos. Photos of the dead may seem very macabre. But for families who have endured the loss of stillbirth, they may be the only physical proof they have that their child really did exist and wasn't just a figment of a morbid nightmare.

Even in the midst of coping with the emotional annihilation, there were critical decisions to be made, decisions we did not feel prepared to make. We had to decide on burial or cremation. We had to tackle the task of choosing a casket. We had to pick a funeral home to orchestrate the service.

Stillbirth attacks the family in many ways. Obviously, there is emotional and physical trauma, but there is also a financial burden. While this is an intensely taboo subject, the financial cost of stillbirth should be addressed here. In addition to sometimes astronomical medical costs, families must pay funeral home costs, whether a child is buried or cremated. If parents choose to bury their baby, there is the cost of a burial plot. A casket or urn must be purchased, which can vary from relatively inexpensive to high-end. A headstone must be purchased, an item that can run the gamut in price. A minister must be paid to officiate at the funeral service itself. Then there are costs for a reception hall, if you choose to gather after the service. If you serve food, add that cost to the list. All these expenses can compound an immense burden at an already difficult time.

Before leaving the hospital, we were given a total of exactly four pamphlets as resources for dealing with the grief and loss of our baby. The pamphlets were Dick-and-Jane simplistic basics on dealing with death. I found one of them to be mildly helpful, but it included only small sections by people who had actually experienced the loss of stillbirth. The rest were written in a clinically professional manner. One of the pamphlets I found to be cruelly offensive because it assumed the woman can have another child, while falsely and coldly stating that a new pregnancy would restore feelings of self-worth and confidence. Heading home from the hospital, we had empty arms and broken hearts. To make things harder, I had leaky breasts and we still had to face the nursery, fully decorated and stocked for our baby's arrival.

For a while, I really couldn't even figure out how to function. I felt like there were reminders of my pain at every turn: pregnant women everywhere, babies in shopping carts. It seemed like every commercial on television either was a product for an infant or had a baby in it. I felt as if my world had ended; I simply could not grasp how the rest of the world was able to continue on normally, as if nothing tragic had occurred. As far as my husband and our marriage, it was treacherous to be responsible for trying to hold a relationship together while grieving the loss of our son. It is a truism that everyone grieves in different ways, but that rang true for us. I didn't know how to go on, and it took me a long time to figure it out. Steve says, "For me, going back to the reality of work was an escape from the reality of the loss of our son. It gave me time during the day when I didn't have to think about him." Shock, denial, bargaining, guilt, anger, depression, and finally acceptance and hope are the stages of grief, and we each had to make our way through the stages in our own time.

Even though we felt lost in our own personal hell, we were stunned to discover we were not alone and that stillbirth is very common. We learned that roughly twenty-six thousand pregnancies end in stillbirth each and every year in the United States. We had foolishly lived in a delusion, believing that stillbirth was not a regular occurrence unless you were too poor to receive proper prenatal care. It was startling to learn that a baby is stillborn approximately every twenty minutes, and to parents from all backgrounds and walks of life. Once it happened to us, we learned of many others who had endured the same tragedy. So many people we personally knew had suffered in silence without ever mentioning their own loss, until we too joined the club. All too often, stillbirth is a loss shrouded in silence.

We endured stupid comments made by well-intentioned people: "It's for the best," "You can always have another," and "How would you like us to dispose of the remains?" We had friendships that proved strong enough to endure our tragedy and others that ended because people didn't know how to deal with our son's death. Our friends and family learned that when it comes to helping someone through the loss of a stillborn child, just being there when needed is what matters.

We attended a grieving parents' support group to help us through our journey toward healing. I designed and created a cross-stitch memorial in honor of our son. It is framed and hung prominently in our home. It proudly displays Steve Anthony II's name and birth date above a delicate angel that is sleeping on a cloud.

After Steve II's death, we were told over and over, "Time heals all wounds." But I don't believe that time can heal the loss of a child. Losing a child leaves a gaping hole in your heart and dreams. Eventually, time does scab over the wound so it does not bleed or hurt all the time and you learn to amend your dreams. But on holidays and what would have been milestones in our son's life, the scab breaks back open just a little bit. It's just not as excruciating as it was in the beginning. In fact, we recently paused to note that he would be getting his driver's license this year, if he had lived.

Initially, I spent substantial amounts of time crying at his grave. I had been taught to believe there was a natural order to life, and my son dying before me seemed like a direct violation of that order. Christmases were spent decorating a tiny tree that we placed near his headstone. The tree, complete with battery-operated lights and decorations, infuriated the memorial garden because it was a direct violation of the rules and regulations regarding winter grave decorations. At first, it was hard to find a way to integrate my son's dying into our living. I personally was not able to make the leap from grieving to healing until we moved across the country, a year and a half after the loss of Steve II.

And it wasn't until I made it into this healing stage that our marriage really began to function as a couple, with a "we" instead of a "me" and a "him."

We had a lot to learn, especially patience, because it took us different amounts of time to make it through the grieving process. We learned to seek out and grasp any small or simple joy. We learned to be around people and not seclude ourselves. We learned to allow ourselves time alone. We learned to talk about our emotions. We learned to seek out support groups when needed. We learned all of these things from a child who never even took a breath. Our son taught us so much.

We are now able to talk about all the positive ways our son helped change and shape our family. After recovering from the initial loss, we decided we wanted another child. We knew we desperately wanted to be parents, and we embarked on a nearly decade-long journey to become parents again.

After Steve II, we tried to conceive naturally. However, it was to no avail. I suffer from a condition called polycystic ovarian disease; our son's conception had been a miraculous, spontaneous, natural pregnancy. That miracle was not repeated, much to our sadness.

We were frustrated that we had to go to such extreme efforts, but the parental urge still nagged louder. We decided to try infertility treatments. The doctor had us try planned intercourse, every other day. When planned intercourse didn't work, the doctor prescribed fertility medications. When medications didn't work, intrauterine inception (IUI) was attempted, a procedure in which sperm is injected directly into the uterus during ovulation. When IUI didn't work, we tried in vitro fertilization (IVF).

The initial news of the IVF implantation was good. My husband and I were told we were once again expecting a child. However, at only 6 weeks' gestation, an ultrasound revealed the fetus was no longer viable and a dilation and curettage (D & C) was required.

Steve still wanted to try to conceive a biological child. I, however, was no longer willing to endure fertility treatments. I came to the resolution that I no longer wanted to try for a child that would be ours genetically. I decided that adoption was the new route we should consider, because I did not want to remain childless.

We carefully researched adoption through both private and international agencies. They all wanted ludicrous amounts of money, in my opinion—much more than we could afford. I wanted to raise and love a child, not buy one. Luckily, we found out about public adoptions through our state. We were scared about the possibility of getting our hearts broken, but proceeded with the licensing required by the state.

In November of 2002, we received a call asking if we would like to meet a sixteen-month-old Hispanic boy. He had been removed from his parents' care when he was ten months old. The state had taken him due to parental mental health issues, as well as parental drug use, homelessness, neglect, and possible child abuse. The boy's biological father was in prison and had never shown interest in parenting. The child's mother had six previous children, all of whom had been removed by the state and placed for adoption. The state wanted to place him in a permanent home, with the intention of the family adopting him. When we arrived at the foster home, the door opened, and there crouched a very small boy, nervously peering out from behind the couch at us. He was so small and needy; I couldn't wait to hold and love him.

The state required that the child be transitioned from his current foster home into our household. Transitioning meant that the first few times we were allowed to see him, we met at his current home. During the next few visits, we were allowed to take him on outings. Continuing the process, we were allowed to bring him to our home for a short stay, the next step toward moving him home with us.

On the night before our ninth wedding anniversary, another social worker called, asking if we would be interested in meeting another child, a six-week-old African American baby boy. Even though we had begun the transition process with one child, we decided we were anxious to meet this infant, too.

This second child's biological father was unknown. The child's mother was unprepared to parent and was willing to relinquish all her rights so he could be adopted quickly. He was born with a rare disorder called fetal hydantoin dilantin syndrome. This syndrome is an effect of a medication that his biological mother had to take for grand mal epileptic seizures during her pregnancy.

The appointment was scheduled for the following morning, the day of our anniversary. The moment I saw him from across the room, I fell head over heels in love. He was so little. He had a huge smile. His body was stuck in a reversed arch position, his muscles locked tight, due to the syndrome from which he suffered.

When the little one was placed in our arms, we knew instantly that we had received the perfect anniversary gift. We were meant to nurture this child also. When the social worker asked if we were interested in adopting the child, we boldly replied, "Yes. When can we take him home?"

This child was an infant, so no transition was needed. The social worker promptly went to the courthouse and had the judge approve the process, granting us immediate custody. We started the day simply celebrating our anniversary. We completed it with one child in our arms and another soon to come home.

Less than one week after we brought our infant son home, our older child's transition was completed ahead of schedule. As parents, we took off running. We went from having no children and a desperate need to be parents, to having a sixteen-month-old and a six-week-old, both of whom had special needs. And we loved every single minute of it.

Our older adopted son was diagnosed as developmentally delayed. He had a complete distrust of people and would hide from most. We endured supervised, weekly one-hour visits with his schizophrenic biological mother. The state ended visits with her only four months after we brought him home. He bonded with my husband during the transition period; however, he did not immediately bond with me. Initially, in fact, he was terrified of all women. Psychological evaluations revealed the lack of bonding was because he was suffering from emotional trauma caused by situations he faced early in life. I had to wait patiently for this child to be ready to accept my affection toward him.

Our younger son had a myriad of medical issues. We knew he would require a lot of care and patience, but we were ready for the job. He needed extensive physical therapy as an infant because of his muscular issues. Not only did he need weekly physical therapy visits, but his therapy also required us to help him perform more than twenty exercises, three times daily, at home. We tackled the therapy with vigor. We created patty-cake-type games for the exercises, so that it would not seem like painful therapy for our infant. Our baby was developmentally delayed and had neurological disorders and severe asthma. He required occupational therapy, pulmonology appointments, and gastroenterology appointments. His medical issues read like a grocery list, but we tackled his special needs with enthusiasm and dealt with them while he was young.

Our stillborn son, Steve II, had created in us an aching need to be parents, to have a child to hold. We were willing and happy to handle issues that others might not have been able to fathom. We openly admit we may be overprotective because of the loss of our son, Steve II, but we also believe that we have more patience with our living children because of him. We have witnessed many parents lose patience or show irritation at diaper changes, late-night feedings, or middle-of-the-night ear infections, while we enjoyed these parental duties. We have lost a child, so any duty we get to perform is a privilege, not a burden; we know what the alternative could be. Our biological child taught us that children are a privilege and a blessing. He taught us the pain of loss. In large part because of Steve II, we are able to relish our duties. We eat dinner together, and we take the time to find out the best and worst parts of our children's days, a routine they look forward to.

With intensive therapy and unconditional love, our children have flourished. They no longer require intense medical interventions. Both now seem like typical, happy, and well-adjusted children. In fact, you would never know that they had been classified as having special needs when they were young. Both boys are active and intelligent. One is shy, and the other a social butterfly. The boys, now ages seven and eight, have always been aware that they are adopted. When asked about their adoptions our older one recites, "We are special because our Mommy and Daddy chose us." The younger smiles and says, "I grew in my Mommy's heart, not her tummy."

The boys are also aware that they had an older brother who died. We have taken trips back to Wisconsin with the boys to visit their big brother's grave. They have curiously questioned us about his passing and their own mortality.

I believe our stillborn son changed the direction of our lives, as well as the lives of our adopted children and family. Seventeen years after the loss of our son, we are able to smile when we talk of him and see all the positive changes that were created by his short life. I once heard a saying, by an unknown author, that summed up my son's life: "He did so much to be so little, but angels always do!"

My husband Steve says, "I know it may sound odd, but I would not change what happened with our son. He helped to make us who we are today. He helped shape and define the amazing life that we have, and for that I am grateful." I believe our son taught us that, even though it feels like it, loss is not the end. In fact, it may very well be the beginning.

CHAPTER SEVEN

Mothering Grief

Angie M. Yingst

I sometimes have the urge to just go to the place reserved for particularly disturbing sixties films where the distraught mother loses all touch with reality and dresses a porcelain doll in her baby's clothes and calls it by her dead child's name. I would surround myself with all things Lucy—her hair, her picture, the little baby doll that I bought for her Christmas, her ashes. I could create a fancy Victorian museum out of all her things. I would wear long black veils, wrap myself in another reality, and rock in the corner. The neighbor children would dare each other to walk in front of the house, peek at my bedroom window, and speed home on their bikes. I would weep until I believed she was alive again. It would be morbid and ugly, but somehow deeply satisfying. But I have a living, breathing child who needs me. Even if I retreated for just one day, I fear I would go fully insane and never return to my beautiful life.

When asked how many children I have, I change my answer depending on the situation. Sometimes, when I just don't want to break a stranger's heart, I allude to only one. "Beatrice is standing over there," I point. But in my heart, and everywhere else, I have two daughters. One is standing over there, and the other is in a heartbreakingly small urn on an antique secretary in my living room. I say it out loud sometimes: "I have two daughters. Two beautiful daughters." It sounds like a wish.

I am a healthy thirty-six-year-old woman mothering a two-year-old and a dead baby. My second daughter died in utero at 38 weeks of pregnancy, and I didn't know it. I went about the day wondering when I last felt her move. And then I was listening to my belly with my husband's stethoscope, not really thinking anything could be wrong. And then I became terrified. And then I thought, "Maybe she is dead." And then she was dead. It wasn't a change of reality, but of perception. I will never know the moment of my daughter's last heartbeat, but I will always remember the moment when I last thought she could be alive. I crossed over from my naïve, oblivious, the-world-is-mostly-a-just-place land into a new horrible alternate dimension where my baby dies. Even though this life, my friends, my house, and my family look the same, they are completely different.

Stillbirth had always seemed so Victorian to me—something that happened to people in another era, another time, because of inadequate citrus intake and bloodletting. But it happened to me after I had two healthy, uneventful pregnancies. I am a modern woman with tattoos and good health insurance whose daughter was stillborn for no medical reason whatsoever. We opted to find out everything and anything about her death. We performed autopsies, blood tests, chromosomal studies, and genetic counseling. They told us nothing more than what we already knew: she died. She was perfectly healthy, just dead.

For many months after she was stillborn, I would wake up forgetting Lucy had died. Confused by the dawn, I would think she was still just waiting to be born. At seven on a Sunday night, I went into the hospital frightened by her lack of movement. I came home at eleven on Monday night without a baby, a deflated empty belly, postpartum hemorrhoids, engorged breasts, and a broken heart. In the early days, I wanted to write Post-it notes to myself, like my grandmother in her old age, so I wouldn't be caught off guard as I reached for my stomach:

> Your daughter is dead.
> You realized yesterday she is not coming back.
> You put away her clothes except for those beautiful fuzzy socks that you bought her for Christmas. You did that on purpose.
> Lucy had your nose.
> You saved a picture of her in a hidden folder on your computer, so you don't happen upon it. The folder is labeled "Christmas."

I experienced her death all over again each morning of those early months. I would cry and remember the ultrasound without movement. The darkened room where she was birthed. Then Beatrice would call me from her room, "Mama. Mama." She is waiting to be mothered, seemingly unaware of the person missing from our family. I admit that I appreciate my living daughter in a way I didn't before Lucy died. I run my fingers through her hair and think, "How did you make it here? How is it that you lived so easily? All you have to do is eat and breathe, poop and giggle." I get to hold one of my children every day. But not Lucy. I still don't have her in my arms. I mother a child that looks exactly like the child who died and is passing milestones my dead baby will never pass. Glorious acts of normalcy. Kisses and the first unprovoked "I love yous." It is strange to have a toddler remind you of your dead newborn baby. I imagine if Lucy lived, people would coo at her, "She looks like Beatrice." But now, I look at Beatrice some mornings and think, "She looks like Lucy."

Life never stopped for us. There wasn't a pause button where I could grieve, then return to oblivious toddlerdom. No one came to watch our daughter while we keened. We tag-teamed; when I was too distraught, my husband became the rock, and I took over when my husband couldn't manage. I take care of my beautiful living daughter, yes, who had no idea that I was so sad that I wanted to turn into a thousand pieces of ash and let the wind carry me in all the directions closer to oblivion. I have a daughter who needs me to get up and get her milk whether I am sobbing or not, who still wants snacks, games, and heartbreaking children's songs about babies falling out of trees and monkeys going to heaven in a little rowboat.

As a stay-at-home mother, I see the cadre of women in sweatpants at the playground, the checkout people at the market, the coffeehouse barista, and the librarian as my coworkers. We make chitchat around the proverbial water cooler. Story time is like a staff meeting with lattes, discreet texting, and nods of acknowledgment. A surprisingly large amount of my time in public is spent making small talk. After Lucy died, I holed up in our Fortress of Solitude for months. I imagined that every place I once thoughtlessly patronized had a person stationed at the front door just waiting to bombard me with questions about our new baby—or worse, with questions that had nothing to do with our loss. Suddenly, small talk seemed so impossibly cruel.

"How are you?"

"What have you been up to?"

Crying? Mourning? Cursing God? Finding meaning in this world? There is no answer that does justice to my daughter. Mostly I just sort of smiled and said, "Not much." I immediately apologize to Lucy, a Hail Mary under my breath. "I'm sorry, love, you are much more than chitchat to me." I always feel like this half-smiling woman is waiting for more small talk–type information. But speaking of the death of your child gives any conversation the kind of *gravitas* that is unwarranted at the butcher shop. As they walk away, I want to call after them, tugging Beatrice hopelessly behind me. "I also grieve," I want to say. "I had a baby who died. She was six pounds. Nineteen inches long. I wail into my pillow during the whole of Bea's naptime now. We do crafts every day to forget for a moment that she isn't here. And I write before the sun comes up. I clean up spilled milk without crying. I do laundry. Walk the dog. Play pat-a-cake. Pretend that my older daughter didn't lose a sister with whom she should be doing these activities. I recite the same damned children's book fifteen times a day with forced enthusiasm. Hide my insomnia under layers of coffee. I sing songs about spiders and stars. And I am unbelievably sad."

I like the version of me people tell me about. The brave person. The strong wife. The wise sage. The sane friend. The good mother. I can see myself steeling myself and being brave against the evil gnarly-fingered image of Death pointing at my womb, as his companions Grief and Hopelessness wait in the wings chewing their nails impatiently. I am two separate mothers: a creative, loving, compassionate, strong mother, and a broken, sad, bereaved mother. I am not curled in a fetal position most days; Bea won't allow me to do that. I have actually paid my bills on time every month since Lucy died. I go to the market every week, do laundry, write pages upon pages of journal entries in the early morning before my daughter wakes, even take Beatrice to the playground. Does this make me a strong, brave, good mother? I sometimes think bravery and strength, the attributes with which people often describe babylost mothers, connote that this life was a choice.

I would have chosen a different path for myself. A simple one. I would have chosen an easy birth, a live child, a quick latch, and a good sleeper. I would have chosen to be blissfully ignorant of how much a baby-size urn costs, of what my husband's worst moment looks like, and of reading in an autopsy report how much my dead daughter's heart weighs. I choose to be present and whole for my daughter. Yes, I guess I am strong some days. What about the days those people don't see me? Where we watch every *Harry Potter* movie in a row, curled up together on the couch eating snacks? Am I brave and strong then? What about those days when I can't manage to pull it together, and I call my sister to take my daughter and I sob all day? Sometimes I want to explain that I am not brave or strong, I am simply polite. I don't even know how else to be. I was raised to not howl in front of strangers, or even good friends.

When friends, neighbors, and acquaintances do know of our loss, they tell me stories about how their friends are affected by death, stories about a child's sudden illness in their community, tales of disaster, scenes of horrible accidents and senseless tragedies. I sense they are trying to find a connection with me now that I am the embodiment of grief. They start the story like this, "I was thinking about you the other day. A family I know at the daycare lost their four-year-old to the flu. The flu! Can you imagine?"

Yes, unfortunately, I can imagine.

In some ways, I think tragedy and compassion are what I have now. In quite another way, it feels so cruel to keep being reminded how chaotic, random, and brutal the universe is. Realizing that others have it worse than me isn't comforting; I simply want to be the last of the sufferers. A dying breed of the dying breed.

I miss normal conversation. Among the many things I lost when my daughter died, that is one I sort of recognized immediately. "I will always be that woman whose daughter died," I remember saying over and over in the emergency room. After I passed the ubiquitous year mark since her death and birth, I find my grief is not as raw. The pain is not acute. It is right below the surface of everything, easily accessed by the slightest provocation. I have to be mindful that it is easily misplaced and brought out. There is a kind of blunt ennui, misanthropy, and anger. I have become bitter in my grief. Though I was emotionally fragile in the months following Lucy's death, I also felt a lot of compassion for everything. I was an exposed heart. Now I feel like my heart is two sizes too small. So I seek others like me. Other grieving mothers. In this world of talking to other babylost mamas, I feel OK. We talk about television shows, our children, our marriages, doing laundry, and yes, our grief. I feel happy, even. Creative. Normal.

Still, it is hard to talk about my live child around dead-baby mamas, and it is hard to talk about my dead baby around live-baby mamas. It is so complicated, the emotions around having one living daughter and one dead one. I am a mother to both of them—actively a mother to Beatrice and Lucy. Sure, I love Lucy as deeply and completely as I love my Beatrice. That is a given; any mother would understand that. And I ache that she is not here. That pain, I absolutely know, is something only a mother feels. I miss Lucy. I just miss her. I miss the idea of what our family was supposed to be. I miss our future. I think other mothers can empathize with that, too. But what other mothers might not understand is how present Lucy is in our home. She demands, like a living child. "Pay attention to me, Mommy. Pay attention." And I sometimes spend the day in bed sobbing, giving in to her demands. The Lucy-sized hole in our lives sucks our attention. A few months after she died, I asked my two-year-old who Lucy is. Her reply: "Lucy is Mommy crying." Her sister is my grief.

All this mothering and grieving and mothering again, it is an exhausting business. Some days, I am a normal mother, light and carefree, packing a picnic to enjoy the last bits of summer. Other days, I cry when my drink tumbles from my shaking hands. "I can't even keep a glass of water alive," I sob as Bea stares at me, afraid and confused. As much as I celebrate all the ways I am a mother to Beatrice and Lucy, I mourn all the ways I can't be a mother, not just to Lucy, but also to Beatrice. To mother and grieve means I also live with overwhelming guilt—a deep guilt that Beatrice's childhood will echo with the grief and sadness that is now my family's reality. I cannot protect her from loss, no matter how desperately I wish it were different. I will have to have raw conversations about death in such a real, exact way much earlier than I ever anticipated. It makes me shudder. My beautiful, innocent two-year-old daughter will fear her own mortality long before I did.

When guilt does creep into my grief, it is never guilt that I couldn't keep Lucy alive in me. I did the best I could. The best all the books had to offer: no caffeine, no drugs, no drinking. I took my folic acid. I meditated and practiced prenatal yoga. I ate no blue cheese (oh, how I missed you). Instead, I feel a nagging, maternal guilt about Beatrice's childhood and happiness. When I think of a new piece of jewelry with Lucy's name, or tweak the design for my Lucy tattoo, or invent a new way of honoring Lucy, or spend hours on the computer reading other grieving mothers' blogs, I become racked with guilt that I don't do that for Beatrice. I don't read blogs about toddlers. Will Beatrice grow up noticing how all my jewelry, my tattoos, my art, and my writing are about the daughter who is not there?

I teach Beatrice about her sister. She doesn't remember me pregnant with Lucy anymore. I went to the hospital and came back not pregnant. No baby. I talk about Lucy. We look at pictures together. I tell Beatrice that she is a big sister. And yet, I feel like I introduce her to a sister I end up killing in the next breath. "Here is your sister. Isn't she beautiful? She is dead. She will never play with you. She will never run with you. She will never annoy you. She is loved by me. Love her too. Be nice to her. Remember her, even though you never met her."

Complicated. Guilt-ridden. Sad. It is not how I thought I would mother, but sometimes I think all parents and mothers experience these feelings, over different things. I can only hope it guides me into teaching my daughter about impermanence and compassion, giving and listening, appreciating and acknowledging, and most importantly, about love and support. When my daughter reflects on her childhood, I hope she is not afraid of death and loss—that I have given her the ability to sit with someone weeping and just listen. For myself, I can only hope that these years without my daughter help me grow to the greater part of humanity—greater compassion, greater love, and greater life and that it makes me a better mother, wife, human being, and friend. I just wish it were because of any other reason than the death of one of my children.

CHAPTER EIGHT

In a Wild Place

Rachel Graham

Yesterday I planted some hardy snowdrops at our daughter's grave. It would have been her sixteenth birthday. The snowdrops were from the garden of a friend in Scotland, the only person who still acknowledges Laura's special day with us each year, which I appreciate.

Laura died during labor at 40 weeks' gestation. She had fetal distress and was delivered by an emergency C-section immediately after my admission. There was a lot of meconium. No medical reason for her death was ever found; she was perfect.

I was unprepared for a death. I was well prepared for a positive birth and was a bit shocked by the intensity of my first-ever labor pains. I was so huge that I was desperate to give birth. When I came round from the anesthetic and they told me I was fine but we had lost the baby, I didn't comprehend what the words meant. *How can you not find a baby in a maternity hospital?*

After morphine, everything is a bit of a muddle; it was like being drunk at some important event where you are trying not to miss anything. There was a lot of crying going on: my husband in the corner; the midwife, which was touching; and then the first of the visitors. It was our earthquake, and the shock was colossal.

A fresh stillborn baby is beautiful to touch. I was so proud of my daughter; her skin was so smooth and she had a chubby little face. I was overcome by the love of a mother and thought that perhaps she would wake up. Later they would take her away to the mortuary and after that she felt different, like a little frozen chicken with a flat back. They brought her out for visitors—

family and close friends. I wanted everyone to see her. We were encouraged to take photographs, which seemed gruesome at the time but turned out to be very precious later. The pictures proved she was there and real. I washed her and dressed her and changed a nappy-full of meconium. This was amazing because she was my first baby and I had never done these things before. I dressed her in a shawl knitted by a family at work. I took comfort wrapping her in something warm for her cold home.

They put us in a room for two, Robert and me, and that was good. We did a lot of talking with the endless visitors and then cried in between, huddled together and exhausted. The two extremes were so odd—we were either hunched together on the bed with our dreams washed down the gutter, or chatting away happily with our visitors. Little kindnesses went a long way: a hot, milky coffee from the nurse; or busy midwives who would linger and talk, making me feel like they had all the time in the world. We even laughed. The midwives were precious people to us—they had seen her, they had been there.

Going home was a silent nightmare, and in those early days my pillow became a phantom baby. There were a lot of mornings spent in bed opening all the cards, and trips out to buy more vases to hold the flowers that kept arriving. Why was I trying to mop the floor for the funeral guests with an aching wound? Why did I have to have milk when I had no baby? And it came in when I was in the shower, I remember, which was shocking. It came spurting out, taking me by surprise. I didn't know that my milk would come in, and it distressed me. The milk was a cruel reminder that my body thought I had a baby to feed. I looked at myself in the mirror and wailed until Robert came to see what all the noise was about.

Who knows how to plan a funeral? Who should come? Who would acknowledge our baby and who would prefer to forget? How can you celebrate a life unknown to most, but appreciated by a few? I knew her every twist and turn and the endless hiccups in the night. I felt her every kick. But who else knew Laura?

At the baby garden where Manchester buries its infant dead, I realized we were not alone. There are others, too many. In years to come it would become a place of strange comfort. Many of the engraved names became familiar. The way the garden has expanded over the years serves as a grim reminder of the many families who lose their babies.

We have faith and felt early on that Laura was safe. That reassuring thought came the first time Robert went home from the hospital and found that a baby iris had opened in our back garden. Our little girl was called Laura Iris, and this little flower was a little whisper to us that God had seen and understood our grief. Soon a picture came to me in a dream, a picture of Laura with Jesus on the other side of a lake, a mental image that brought me great comfort.

Later, the whole area of faith was harder—much harder—and I struggled and wrestled with God for many months. Eventually, in a dream I was confronted with the choice of quitting and going it alone or sticking with the Lord. I woke up and decided that, even if I didn't understand, I was safer with God. I figured that He didn't make my baby die, but He allowed it to happen. This knowledge was either going to seriously screw me up forever or be the turning point for a new depth in life. It took a lot of reading, talking to people, thinking, and praying to get me to this point. I think Robert always had more of a peace about it, but I wrestled with this great weight for months. It doesn't feel heavy anymore.

Now, I never assume that God is going to make everything turn out just fine, but I know He is going to be there.

During the night Laura died, while Robert sat in a chair by my bed, struggling to come to terms with what had happened, a verse in the book of James came to him: "You have heard of Job's perseverance and have seen what the Lord finally brought about." This suggested to us that if we persevered, God would be able to bring good things out of the bad that had happened to us.

As the months passed, I found that I felt more comfortable than I used to around others in distress. I wasn't afraid to ask questions and listen. Perhaps that was a start.

At first, though, I felt raw, like a grated lemon. I had a wound to hide and I didn't want to be around anything that might cause further pain. I was sensitive to words that others said—or didn't say. I wanted to talk endlessly about our baby. I wanted to show everyone photos. At night, I thought about digging her up. Perhaps I could put her in the pram and walk her around the local streets. Who would know she wasn't alive? I wept with deep sobs such as I had never experienced before and was suddenly overcome in embarrassing places with people who didn't know me well: in the dentist's chair, during a colleague's visit, with the milkman, in the middle of a crowded train. I couldn't trust myself; at any moment I might be overwhelmed.

I felt a bit mad and in a wild place. At night that winter, there was a disturbed teenager who howled along our road, and from my bed I was with him all the way. His aching cries captured the pain of my spirit at that point.

About this time, I discovered SANDS, the stillbirth and neonatal death support charity. On my first visit to the local support group, I was overcome by an avalanche of words that I needed to say to a room of people who understood. As if I sat in a confessional booth, I could admit my madness. And listening to the others there assured me that we all have our own insanities.

It was a cathartic moment, and I felt elated to be among others who had been through what I had, to be able to express my grief fully.

SANDS would continue to be a source of protection to me. In my day-to-day life, I could file away things to share at the next meeting. Nothing was too extreme. As the years passed, I became the old-timer, and my ability to recognize the rawness of others was a sign that I had made progress.

Grieving as a couple was strange. At first we were very close, but somehow we became separated in our lostness. I wanted to cry and talk, but Robert didn't. He wanted to get away from the pain he was experiencing, put his foot to the metal, and accelerate away from the loss. I was upset with him. He was annoyed with me. I took his avoidance as denial; he took my openness as weakness—or so it felt to me. I thought he loved Laura less than I did, and I didn't want to be stopped from crying or made to feel better, because I wanted to hurt.

We got through it, eventually. Years later, he wrote a novel about the grief of a couple who lose a child. I went to SANDS to talk and talk and talk. I think the differences between the ways we each dealt with our bereavement and the process of coming to terms with them strengthened our marriage. It was like a fracture, healing up a bit deformed but thicker, stronger.

Five months later, I was pregnant again.

We were guarded and cautious, afraid to hope for success. I felt afraid and empty inside. I kept it quiet and avoided talking about another baby. Almost to disguise the pregnancy from myself, I wore clothes that were too big for me. I opted for a cesarean section so that my baby wouldn't die in labor. I didn't trust myself. When I went into the hospital to deliver, I didn't take any baby clothes in case we didn't bring her home.

We did, though, and she was lovely, and having a live baby girl was a healing process. This time during the delivery, I was awake and could see her and hear that first yell. She seemed like a miracle. We called her Poppy, which means "my consolation." And she has been. She likes to point out, however, that if Laura had lived she wouldn't have been there at all—but we don't dwell on that one.

We had a son, too. By then, I'd had too many cuts and my womb was thin, so toward the end of that pregnancy, I walked about precariously, as if I might fall apart. He was born three weeks early, for safety. "For safety"—those words are important to me. No risks. I'm not a risk-taker anymore, not with babies, and I have to keep quiet around those who are pregnant, in case I spoil their dreams.

He was white like a little snowman. Being born early, he had that white coating called *vernix caseosa*, which protects the baby's skin from constant exposure to amniotic fluid in the womb. We called him Noah.

Out of this story comes another one, about a little girl lost to her parents and parents who lost a little girl. It happened on Valentine's Day, in China.

Soon after Laura, while our hearts were still sore, we saw a documentary on TV about baby girls in orphanages due to China's one-child policy, and we said to ourselves that one day, because girls seemed so precious, we would adopt one like this. One day.

It was over ten years later that we took a flight to Beijing with Poppy, who was ten, and Noah, who was seven. We were to meet Maisy, who was one, on our second day in China. The night before, I lay in bed in a sweat, thinking how mad we were to be adopting.

We were called straight from a jet-lagged breakfast to a conference room at the hotel—summoned with the words, "Your daughter is waiting for you." How bizarre. When we entered the large space, for some reason there was very little light. We were invited to sit on the leather executive chairs and there she was, under the table, and she was friendly and mischievous and affectionate and we all liked each other straight away.

It felt different to me, this meeting a daughter. How did she know I was her new mother? She didn't, of course. It was only over the days and weeks ahead that small bonding activities happened—rocking her to sleep; protecting her from harm; bathing, feeding, and playing with her—and she became my little one. We learned to accept each other, gently.

It's another way to be a mother and I am always aware of the grieving mother in China who aches for her daughter. We can share some of the pain of having lost a daughter. There is pain for both mothers, but I have the joy of Maisy, who has been found and is safe. If we hadn't had Laura, we wouldn't have Maisy, who has enlarged us all.

Over the years, we have seen what the Lord finally brought about: Maisy, of course, but also my involvement with SANDS, where I have been able to give something back; and work that Robert has been doing for many years with young people and the arts. Both of these commitments came directly out of the experience of losing a child. We really have seen how good things have come out of bad.

Last night, as I do every year on Laura's birthday, I lit a candle to burn through the night. By the morning, however, it had gone out. I was glad, because the hardest thing about remembrance candles is having to blow them out.

CHAPTER NINE

Born, Again

Meng Kiat Tan

July 27, 2007: They did not find a heartbeat.
July 29, 2007: He was born, still. And she died.

She remembers that day vividly. The details of it had been tattooed into her skin, in ink invisible to all but her. In fact, the ink whispers and sings to her in her dreams. Every week, she scrubs herself over vigorously, and then she smoothes oil over the newly revealed skin. But the details of that day, they never slough off.

She remembers that day, the sick feeling of the surrounding air snapping her like a whip and strangling her. How she had gasped, choked, and held on to herself as the shock threatened to shatter her to pieces.

She remembers that day, when their midwife did not find a heartbeat.

She was told to get on her hands and knees. Perhaps the heartbeat was just hiding—no heartbeat. The midwife then tried a different Doppler, a better one. And still there was silence—no heartbeat.

So they drove to the hospital.

"No, no heartbeat. Nothing. Call Dr. W. and let him know to come in."

She watched the nurse's lips move as she uttered those words, and tried to imagine that those shapes her lips made were other words and meant different things.

But those words meant what they meant. Her son's heart had stopped beating. His life had ended while in utero.

The door closed. With no possibilities for negotiations.

And then another door opened, and she had to go through, even if she knew not what was beyond. She saw only darkness lurching toward her.

First, her baby needed to be born. It took two days of repeated coaxing before her body realized that the baby needed to be born. Those two days were hard work. She walked and walked—an exercise rumored to aid in the baby's descent. She squatted. She walked some more. She braced, she paced, she wore a path between bed and door.

Her body yielded, eventually. With her eyes shut tight, shrieking in pain, and still pregnant with disbelief, she gave the final push to bring her baby out into this mortal world.

This cannot be happening, she silently pleaded. *Please let this be a mistake. He is going to cry, we are going to hear a baby's cry and know that it was all just an atrocious mistake.*

But it was no mistake. He was born still, and silent.

Nonetheless, his small body, with its remnant warmth from being in his mother's womb, was immediately placed upon her belly; she saw his face for the first time and touched him for the very first time. Oh, he looked so much like his two older sisters! Those long fingers, those awkward long toes, the flat nose, and the dark blob of hair. There was to be no mistake; his features spoke of an intimate relationship to his siblings.

For several hours after, she held him, cradling him close, burning to imprint the weight and shape of her baby's body against her bosom. She sang to him, lullabies familiar, in a voice that threatened to crack on every note. She stroked his smooth cheeks, and dabbed his exposed skin with cotton pads soaked with saline solution. You see, his sisters had yet to arrive at the hospital to meet him, but he was already beginning to change, rapidly. Life is transient, fragile, and a determined follower of rules. Once the breath of vitality is gone, the body begins its journey back to earth. (She thought of Snow White lying pretty in that glass coffin for days, untainted skin soft and rosy—an outrageous lie!) His skin was darkening and shriveling, surrendering moisture to the cold still air of the room. She witnessed, in sped-up time lapse, how one ages, how life drains away, how a body wizens. It was not a pretty sight, but there was a bizarre beauty to this intimate experience of beholding it so clearly, nothing embellished. Texture altered, color changed. No illusions. And so for hours she stood by the threshold of Life and Death, loving him, kissing him, and cried herself a river of bitter regret.

The hours crept by, and soon the veil of night fell. And it started to rain.

Despite the rain, the man from the mortuary kept his word and appeared in her room to take her son away, to prepare for his cremation. It was time to say good-bye. It was time to acknowledge that she and her son stood on opposing sides of that threshold. She was exhausted after two days of labor, giving birth, and holding him, but she wished to hold him longer—there is nothing like the wonderful weight of a small package in one's arms when it is a baby. It did not matter that she already had two daughters. The tenderness and heartache of holding him only intensified, especially when the time she had was so limited. Especially when Death refused to look back.

The man from the mortuary stepped solemnly into her room. He was tall, big, bald, and silent. He spread a Winnie-the-Pooh blanket on the hospital bed and told her she could lay her baby on it. Suddenly everyone in the room (the mother, the father, the baby's sisters, the nurses—but not the man) began to cry and shake; wet, salty tears splashed onto shoulders and ran down innocent cheeks. Outside, the rain fell, sheets of shredded white.

She set her son on the blanket; it took so much strength to put him down. She kissed him, one more time—one last time. Then the man from the mortuary stepped forward and quietly wrapped the blanket over and around him. Over and around, for the baby had no need for air. He knew the motions well, and despite the keening around him, he did not fumble—he was calm, quiet, and sure. Then the wrapped-up bundle was picked up, put on the man's shoulder, and carried away. He walked through the door; he did not look back.

How she burned to chase after the man and beg him to please give her back her son. Instead she simply collapsed and cried some more. And with each sob and every heaving breath, she slowly died. The man had walked away not just with her son; he was also walking away with her family's dreams, their hopes and fantasies.

> But human beings have a soul which lives forever, still lives after the body is turned to dust. The soul goes climbing up through the clear air, up till it reaches the shining stars. Just as we rise up out of the sea and look at the countries of human beings, so they rise up to beautiful unknown regions—ones we shall never see.

So said the old grandmother of the littlest mermaid in Hans Christian Andersen's fairytale "The Little Mermaid." She read that to her daughters and told them that she believed their baby brother must be a star-traveler. That was why they named him Ferdinand: the "ardent voyager." He was a star traveler, spreading his dust around the galaxies.

She believed in souls. She believed in reincarnation. And she also believed in the eternity of dust. Ferdinand is dust. Ferdinand is soul. Both are fluid, morphing, indestructible, elusive, ubiquitous, and eternal.

Cradling these beliefs in her heart, she began to watch intently and listened with heightened attention. A fawn came by their cabin a few times and she wondered, *Is that Ferdinand?* A moth or a butterfly would flutter by, and she silently asked, *Is that you visiting, my son?* As she lay awake in bed on so many nights, forming phantom shadows on walls, ceilings, and doors, she pricked her ears up as she whispered, "Are you there?"

She did not believe that his death meant an end. The thread that was his continued to warp and weft out of the fabric of their family life. His older sisters included him in their drawings and talked about him often. When they raised their eyes to the skies, their bodies enfolded by darkness, they sought out the star that may be his home, or perhaps *is* him. The pain and shock of losing him continued. She could not stop wondering why he made the decision to not come earth-side. She could not stop wondering if his soul was still close by. She could not stop wondering if he might perhaps be reborn as another child, into their family again.

> On the ashes of this nest
> Love wove with deathly fire
> The phoenix takes its rest
> Forgetting all desire.
>
> After the flame, a pause,
> After the pain, rebirth.
> Obeying nature's laws
> The phoenix goes to earth. . . .
>
> And one cold starry night
> Whatever your belief
> The phoenix will take flight
> Over the seas of grief
>
> To sing her thrilling song
> To stars and waves and sky
> For neither old nor young
> The phoenix does not die.

—May Sarton (1912–1995)[1]

Some weeks after Ferdinand's death, this poem landed in her mailbox, sent by a friend who told her, "I read this and thought of you."

It was the first time she had encountered the poem, and as her eyes flew over the lines, she began to quiver and howl. The poem made her realize that for weeks she had been a walking corpse: a dead person with a beating heart. She had drawn away from friends and people, intentionally withdrawing into the dark, retreating into a cave. But she did not realize that it was to await a rebirth, or that rebirth was even a possibility.

Nine months after Ferdinand died, she fell pregnant again. *Perhaps Ferdinand's soul is rejoining our family*, she thought.

As the weeks progressed and her belly grew, so did the fears. She had learned that there were a million reasons why babies can die. She questioned whether lightning could strike, once again. And will Death beat Life to the door one more time? She considered the potentiality of seeing Ferdinand's soul again, in a different body, and that gave her courage to plod on despite the gnawing trepidation that she might once again hear only silence and be informed that there was no heartbeat.

One day she laid her hands on her belly and knew viscerally that this soul was not Ferdinand's. She felt deeply that his was never meant to be earth-bound but was destined to be an itinerant soul, traveling amidst realms unknown. It was a bittersweet moment of clarity and acceptance, knowing that his soul, bright and free, was not hers to hold.

She began to buy things for the new little baby, acts of courage and defiance, for she could no longer believe things occur as planned. They still had boxes stuffed with clothes that were for Ferdinand; some still had tags attached and some he would have outgrown had he been born alive. She laundered and folded little baby girl clothes, a campaign for hope to stay. They took out the car seat that was to have been Ferdinand's, and washed it and lifted it, trying to imagine how much more effort would be required to carry it with a baby sleeping in there. (How much does the memory of a dead little baby weigh? Do they gain weight and stature as the years go by?)

One day, a wise old woman whom she did not know very well told her, "Your daughter is the same soul as your son."

She did not understand the riddle. What did the old woman mean? Could she see into the mysterious realm that all babylost parents wish to see? Had she made a mistake in feeling so certain that this new baby's soul was not that of Ferdinand?

The questions filled her head as she awaited the day of the new baby's arrival. Like the phoenix, she groomed her feathers (gingerly), stretched her wings (charily), and then squinted (warily) at the shades of dark in her cave.

Darkness enveloped, light penetrated. In cracks around the entrance (and exit) of the cave she saw the light, thin but sure, slicing at the darkness.

She waited, knowing that was all she could do. Time had no handle she could crank, and though her eyeballs wished to leap out of their sockets to look around the corner, all she could do was wait. Will the time come? Will the baby come to meet her? Will she leave the tangled nest? How long till the heart, all guarded now, can slam uninhibited in its cavity, beating wildly with joy? All she could do was allow time to unfold and for the baby to decide her own journey.

And the baby came, swiftly. Like a decisive and determined storm it vigorously gathered speed; she was pounded with contractions that allowed only hair's-breadth moments of exhalation, with little respite.

"Everything is fine. Baby is fine, heartbeat is fine." She heard her midwife's sing-song assurance, "She is OK, her heartbeat is strong."

How she managed to have heard those words through a bubble, she did not know. She was in a bubble that was suspended in the past and present superimposed. She was birthing again, she realized. Different hospital, different room, the sands of time had shifted, but everything felt so familiar, and even smelled the same. She froze, afraid to break that bubble. What if she moved and the bubble burst and all was lost? She held still, her eyes closed so darkness surrounded her.

The force of Birth, like that of Death, cannot be held back. The baby's head crowned, and she paused to reach down and touch her head: moist, warm, and sticky. Tangible. She could feel the throbbing that was Life. She could even smell Life already—a potpourri of blood, warmth, and vernix.

"You need to listen to me. The baby's shoulder is stuck. No time for whining now. I need you to push, harder."

There was the midwife's voice again. This time her voice rang with urgency. She understood the implications of those words and she pushed. Hard. She felt her bones were going to break and splinter. But she kept pushing. Hard. Eyes shut tight, howling and shrieking like a banshee, she pushed, and the baby was unstuck, and born. She opened her eyes and looked. Light flooded the room.

The baby cried, and so did she. Birth, and rebirth.

Once again, a baby was laid on her belly, and it felt like she had given birth to Ferdinand all over again. Except this time, the baby was warm and squirmy, alive and crying, jostling the air molecules into a frenzy with her little fists punching into the air and her cries jabbing the atmosphere, and everything crackled.

The baby looked exactly like Ferdinand, features familiar, an almost replica. Her expression reminded her of how Ferdinand had looked when she held him for those few hours. Their resemblance startled her. She suspected that she was looking at the new baby through a warped lens, except she clearly knew that she was not. She began to understand why that old woman had said, "Your daughter is the same soul as your son." It was because the soul is fluid and mysterious. It was because both she and her brother were born from the same source, from the undying and fervent yearning for Life.

Lyra Phoenix was born in January 2009, eighteen months after the death and birth of her brother. (Nine months twiced. Nine months to breed the courage to try again; another nine months to navigate the journey out of the labyrinth dark.)

Her birth was her brother Ferdinand's too, again, as the reincarnation of hope and love.

Her birth was her mother's too—a rebirth. Born as a mother of not three, but four children. Born as a mother who understood that Love transcends all boundaries. Born, with a heart that overflows with joy and gratitude: a heart that also has an eternal hole in it, whistling with a sorrow that understands joy.

January 9, 2009: Lyra Phoenix was born.
Her mother was re-born, and
her brother was born too, again.

CHAPTER TEN

Just One Family

Jenell Williams Paris

Mothers in a Brazilian slum don't grieve when their babies die. In Bom Jesus de Mata, a newly bereaved mother may shrug it off or even go dancing. She explains herself easily, "What else can you expect from an angel?" A small, weak, or ill infant is seen literally as an angel, a guest who by definition will visit for only a short time. A mother may even hasten death by denying food and medical care, meager as both are. No official record is taken of the birth or death of slum babies; to the Brazilian state, as well as to mothers, they are not quite human.

When newly arrived Peace Corps worker Nancy Scheper-Hughes became distraught over a baby's death, the mother laughed at her.[1] As intrigued as she was disturbed, Scheper-Hughes left and returned later as an anthropologist to understand death without weeping. Most women in Bom Jesus birth ten, twelve, or more babies but raise only a remnant to adulthood. In the absence of birth control, prenatal care, adequate food, and clean water, a woman expects to lose many babies herself and to witness the same for her neighbors, sisters, aunts, nieces, and daughters. Scheper-Hughes says low expectations for infant survival distort maternal love, trust, affection, and grief. Loving those babies less who are likely to die is a coping mechanism that helps women carry on with their responsibilities to the living. And it's a brutal but shrewd survival strategy to invest despairingly inadequate food and medical care in older children and in babies more likely to live. (Absenteeism is the favored coping strategy for fathers; extreme poverty wreaks havoc on the bonds between lovers, too.)

In a Minnesota suburb, distant from Bom Jesus by both miles and privilege, my expectations ballooned along with my belly. In a wealthy nation with abundant food and medical care, I presumed a healthy gestation, birth, and long life for each baby I conceived. Even when assisted reproductive technology yielded a small litter of zygotes, I believed a meticulous prenatal regimen would swing the odds in my favor. Both of us well-educated professionals with supportive families, my husband and I drew on all our personal and intellectual resources to make the best choices for our triplets. When I passed a milestone week, my obstetrician said, "Things are looking good. You're going to keep these babies!" Losing one or two fetuses was still a terrible possibility, but the likelihood of losing all three faded away with the first trimester.

Feeling my water break during the night in the wrong month, then, was a rude awakening in more than one way. We rushed to the hospital where our obstetrician said, "This is the worst-case scenario. We have to end this pregnancy now." All three placentas were raised and inflamed like cuts; the babies were swimming in infected waters due to a rare uterine infection called chorioamnionitis. To save my life, we would induce labor. We couldn't save theirs; perfectly formed but weighing less than a pound each, the triplets were too premature to live outside the womb. I negotiated with the doctor: if I let the pregnancy go for a few more days, maybe they could reach viability, even if I were to die. I appealed to my husband: if I just let the pregnancy go until the babies and I died together, that would at least allow them a few more days of life. I begged with God: if I birth these babies today, please let them live.

The babies didn't dicker; they followed the orders of the labor-inducing medication, lining up to emerge in sequence. They dropped, boy after boy after boy, into my waiting hands like chocolate kisses from a bag. Delicious as they could be, my appetite for them was fully aroused but they began melting away at once. Hemorrhaging caused another emergency for me and I was wheeled away to surgery with the taste of my sons' sweetness still in my mouth. Ian had been born still, and Simon and Gordon spent their final minutes with their father.

At the time, I viewed that day as a Darwinian struggle: the four of us faced a common enemy, but only the strongest survived. For months, I felt ashamed for being the only one living after that pregnancy. I wasn't suicidal. I didn't want to die; I wanted to have died with them, or better yet, instead of them. It's not easy to emerge from a car accident, a burning building, or a multifetal pregnancy in which everyone else dies. Survivor guilt is just what it sounds like: feeling shame for having survived something to which others succumbed. The guilt stems from worries that perhaps you could have done more to save someone, or that maybe you selfishly ignored someone's distress, or worst of all, that you may have clawed your way to daylight at someone else's expense.

Though I hated myself for it, I resumed my daily life. I went to a yoga class about a week after the babies' deaths. I stood before a mirror in *vrksasana*, or "tree pose," balanced on my right leg, resting my left foot against the inside of my right knee, hands overhead. I wobbled—the sudden loss of pregnancy weight had altered my center of gravity. I regained balance and stared at my appearance: sallow skin, puffy eyes and lips, saggy middle, twiggy arms and legs. My breasts were huge, hard, and painful, filled with unexpressed milk. As others in the class carried on, I gave up. I balled up in *balasana* (in English, "child's pose"), face-down with forehead on the ground, chest on tucked-under knees, and quietly bawled. The instructor, Joel, a trim older man, knew about my babies' deaths. After class, he came over and kissed me on the head, whispering, "You showed up. You began."

Around that time, my counselor made a comment about beginning the healing journey. I protested, "I don't want to heal." I wanted healing for my body, to be sure. I'd consider it a blessing if the physical residue of that difficult pregnancy and its demise could be just a pale, smooth scar. Now, six years later, I still don't take for granted the ease with which I eat, walk, and sleep. But if healing in the broader sense means moving on from my triplets, sealing off that loss with a clean scar, then I'll decline. It's not healing I'm after; I'm on a journey toward integration. I want to have just one story of my life, not two parts titled "before the triplets" and "since the triplets." And I want to have just one family, not a first family of deceased children and a second family of living children (since my triplets' deaths, I have birthed three more sons).

Seeing how dire poverty distorts maternal grief in Brazilian slums makes me wonder how wealth warps mourning in my world. We're told to go after the good life, the happiness and material abundance secured by income, investments, and the security that money can buy. Like cancer, fatal accidents, terrorist attacks, and other tragedies, infant loss is an unwelcome reminder of how tragedy barges into the good life, even when shored up by wealth. And so, as quickly as possible, we look away. Some ignore miscarriage, stillbirth, and early infant death altogether, while others give elaborate attention to the moment of death and the days thereafter. Either way, within a few weeks, bereaved parents are often urged to resume their normal lives, and if they can't be happy, at least begin seeking happiness. I curse every well-intended suggestion to get busy, go back to work, take up flower arranging, or, worst of all, have another baby—as if there's a Baby Customer Service that offers new, working models to compensate for the ones that failed. Though I'm busy now with three living sons, they are not replacements for those who were lost; each is singular. My sorrow over my first three sons is total, as is my joy for the living.

The anti-grief, anti-sadness values of my society are encoded even in everyday conversation. Whether it's pets, spouses, or children, we're expected to mention the living and leave the dead behind; in polite conversation, the dead are unmentionable. Being asked the simple question, "How many children do you have?" leaves me tongue-tied. The easiest and most courteous reply is "three," counting only my living children. In a conversation with a stranger this often suffices, but with acquaintances or friends, "three" makes me worry that I've erased my first three sons. But when I tell the whole truth, I risk being seen as someone who has failed to move on. I've tried it; people sometimes begin counseling me or sharing their own tragedies, or they change the subject or even physically retreat.

Women in Bom Jesus, for the rest of their lives after a loss, include both their angel babies and their living children in their family head counts. When asked how many children they have, the typical response is, "Ten, four living" or "Twelve, six living." Their language shows that, despite the absence of immediate grief over death, lost babies are part of their mothers' lives forever. "Ten, four living" is a simple, everyday expression of how maternal bonds are real and lasting. We grieve quickly and forcefully and then move on. They ease into it and let it last.

Instead of simmering in guilt, bereaved Bom Jesus mothers acknowledge it's the babies, not them, who have moved on. They scrounge for a few pennies to purchase a plywood coffin and paint the cardboard lid light blue. With the coffin left unclasped, babies are buried just two feet under the ground so they can more easily fly toward the blue sky. A mother can believe that she was responsive to her baby's needs. She hosted an angel for a time and then released it to heaven.

One woman said to the anthropologist, "Don't pity the infants who died here. . . . Pity us instead. Weep for their mothers who are condemned to live." This isn't survivor guilt, however; it's a lament for the difficulty of poverty and hunger. Seen in another light, of course, the grief and burial practices I've described, while poignant, are severe necessities for people too poor to afford quality coffins or professional burials. Given better resources, things would surely change in the babies' favor, including the cultural interpretation of weak infants as angels and the disregard mothers often show for them.

I attended yoga class regularly in the early months of grief and soon began following along for the entire session. Each class ended with about ten minutes of relaxation in *savasana*, a lovely-sounding Sanskrit word that translates "corpse pose." I lay flat on my back, all my muscles relaxed, arms at my sides with palms raised. Joel led us into relaxation with these words, "Go inside and you will find peace. You will wake up to find yourself renewed, refreshed, and rejuvenated." I found chaos, panic, and despair. My interior life had become like the home of a hoarder or a cat lady—it was scary to go in there. Each time I failed to find peace, hissing filled my ears, "You're a bad mother, bad yoga student, bad person."

As they were for my triplet pregnancy, my expectations were off. I thought if I tried hard, I would find peace right then, within those ten minutes. Renewal, refreshment, and rejuvenation are coming, but it's taking much longer than ten minutes or even ten months. It takes time to go inside every place in my world—my family, friendships, faith, professional life, and so on—and learn how to be the mother of six, three living. It's taken years to revisit the September day when my sons died and literally re-member it—reassemble its meaning—as the day I received a precious and bittersweet gift, not just hours of merciless trauma.

I'm through with the rush to move on. I'm accepting the invitation to move *with*. My family is all together when Ian, Simon, and Gordon rest, and their father, brothers, and I move, in peace.

CHAPTER ELEVEN

"Then Comes the Baby in the Baby Carriage"

Sherokee Ilse

"Sherry and Tommy sitting in a tree. K-I-S-S-I-N-G. First comes love, then comes marriage, then comes Tammy in a baby carriage." (Tommy was an early boyfriend, and Sherry was my childhood nickname.) Ah, dreams of tomorrow, someday, a long way off, when small children prepare to become parents to smaller children.

All of my life, it seems, was some form of preparation for the children I would have someday. I remember reciting these rhymes as we jumped rope and played house in my bedroom, in our blanketed hideouts, and even in our tree forts in the woods. Playing dolls was one of my passions that continued into my sixth-grade year, even though many of my friends had long before packed their dolls away. While the games I played changed over time, the desire to fall in love, get married, and have children persisted. I would often look at how others parented their children, vowing to do it differently, though occasionally I'd see great parenting and make a mental note to model it. Hopes and dreams built early on, tucked away for another faraway day.

Eventually, I found the man of my dreams. Marriage during my senior year of college seemed natural and timely. Interestingly enough, David was even more consciously looking for both a partner and a mother for children. Years later he admitted to me that before he asked me to marry him, he assessed me, my family, and my own mother to determine if, as he put it, "you would be a good mother to the children I hope we have someday."

So when it was time to begin a family after seven years of marriage, we set upon it very excitedly with quite a bit of naïve optimism. When we learned we were pregnant, we spread the news far and wide and looked at each other with a starry-eyed gaze, knowing that a brand-new, long-awaited adventure was about to begin. Twelve weeks into the pregnancy, our hopes were dashed by a miscarriage. This was not supposed to happen. My sister previously had often described me as the luckiest person she ever knew—everything always seemed to go well for me. But not this time. We "untold" the news, cried some, then quickly took the nurse's advice to take care of my health and then try again. The emotions were safely stuffed away.

A year and a half later, after taking temperatures and noting each sexual encounter, we finally found ourselves pregnant again. This time our optimism was tainted with worry and a focus on getting past the twelve-week miscarriage mark. Once that had happened, we again believed naïvely that all would be well. We readied the room with pretty baby colors and decorations, had baby showers, and believed we would soon be parents of a beautiful baby who would bring much fulfillment to our already wonderful lives. I recall dreaming of special moments, like pushing the baby carriage around the lake and dressing him in the outfits I had sewn and the special ones we had bought. One special dream kept floating up in my mind: going to the mailbox and finding letters addressed from my dear Grandma to Master Brennan Ilse. (I did have a feeling it was a boy, and that was the name we had easily agreed on. No girls' names had come to the forefront yet.)

When that fateful day arrived—Tuesday, November 2, 1981—it was fear and worry that brought me to the hospital. Already my innocence was slipping away. It was one day past our due date, but I didn't feel excitement and anticipatory joy. Though I had gone to an ordinary appointment with my midwife the Friday before, over the weekend I hadn't felt much movement. Believing the widely circulated myth that babies slow down right before birth,[1] I did not take this change seriously—a regret I still bear today.

By Tuesday midday, I couldn't take it any longer, so I went in to the hospital because the clinic was closed for lunch. Four "nonfunctioning" machines later, after an exam and an ultrasound, I was told those devastating words no parent wishes to hear: "I fear your baby has died. There is no heartbeat." Where does one go from there? To the deepest pit . . . deeper and darker than the Grand Canyon on a moonless, stormy, windy night. That's where the real nightmare began. I thought I would never, ever feel whole and happy again. And I didn't for a long, long time.

With little staff guidance, though I could see the sadness and compassion in their eyes, and with the inexperience that comes with such a loss, we barely saw our son. We didn't agree to take pictures, and we showed him to no one in our family. We then left the hospital with no blanket, no outfit, no crib card, no mementos of any kind, and no written materials or knowledge of support groups. He wasn't dressed in an outfit or cuddled, as every baby should be. Instead, I was wheeled out the front door with David walking beside me. Our empty arms matched our broken hearts. Meanwhile, our beloved son Brennan left out the back door to the arms of an unknown funeral director.

As a newly bereaved mother, I learned how hard it was to let go of my dreams of Brennan, who could never be replaced by another baby. I wanted *him* and *him alone* at that time. My arms ached for a long time. I spent many hours in my bed, crying my eyes out. I felt so alone, so crazy, and so tired. I dwelled on it every minute of each day and night, wondering how to live through such a devastating experience. David and I talked and talked, and we cried together. He held me close and offered support, but too soon he had to go back to work. As I think about that now, I wonder how hard that must have been—to attempt to try to resume life again. I couldn't do it. Brennan's death rocked my world and I knew it, and I would never be the same again. A good friend suggested that I follow my own advice, the advice I gave to everyone who was upset or angry about something and merely complained: "What are you going to do to change it?" That was the challenge that I needed to begin shifting my dreams from mothering a new baby to mothering a new mission.

Within a month, I began writing a brochure to help others make better decisions. Things needed to change, and I felt compelled to make something positive out of this horrific experience. My other work no longer mattered, nor did my university studies for my MBA. Instead, I quit them all and devoted myself, day and night, to writing a booklet. The booklet turned into a seventy-plus-page book called *Empty Arms*.[2] One of my new dreams was to have this book available in every hospital in America—to offer hugs, support, love, and concrete advice from the heart of a parent to those who, sadly, would come after me.

Empty Arms and our story were featured in the St. Paul newspaper, and then the story hit the wire and was printed in many cities, bringing stacks of letters, orders for *Empty Arms*, and invitations to speak to hospital staff.

Around that same time, I invited some of the parents who wrote to me to help me start a national organization for bereaved families and their caregivers. We knew we had to move our culture from the Dark Ages into a more enlightened period. Families needed to be taught about their options to see, hold, take pictures, dress and undress, bathe, and say prolonged hellos to their babies before rushing to think about autopsies, funerals, and burials—the difficult good-byes. Our team helped pave the way[3] by reaching out to hospitals and other professionals and by designating October as Pregnancy and Infant Loss Awareness Month. We developed letter-writing campaigns to Hollywood producers and actors, asking them to write infant death into shows, which hadn't yet been done. We began holding Walks to Remember and community memorial services. The frenetic actions to change the way losses were handled kept us all busy and fulfilled. And eventually, over time, with much work from many, we did change things for the better.

For the next almost three decades, I spoke at thousands of seminars, conferences, support groups, churches, and schools. I authored, coauthored, and self-published seventeen books and booklets. I started my own company, Wintergreen Press. I was invited to be on national television shows including *Oprah*, as well as on regional and local media. I have traveled all over the United States and the world spreading this mission, seeking to help improve care and support for bereaved parents and families. Professionally, everything in my life changed. In fact, I continue this work, this mission, as I write this—but I also played the role of mother to two babies who died and subsequently two sons who lived (Kellan and Trevor), followed by an ectopic pregnancy (Bryna) after Trevor.

Yes, my dreams had changed. I no longer focused on being Brennan's new mommy. Instead I was mothering a process—a process of healing myself, reaching out to help others, and finding ways to honor and keep our son's memory and little life alive. This mission has defined a large portion of my life for almost thirty years now.

Thankfully, over the years, I was able to push those baby carriages with living babies inside. And I also had a family mission that helped us release old dreams and seek new ones, including how to keep our baby's memory alive, mark family life milestones, and remember birthdays, while enjoying life with our sons Kellan and Trevor.

As Brennan's first birthday approached I worried and fretted about what I would do. Being someone who seeks control when I can, I decided that having a plan was better than letting the day arrive and evolve. I was nervous and highly emotional as the day drew near.

I called a friend who I knew would support my crazy idea for remembering Brennan's birthday. However, I didn't quite dare tell David. I knew that if he even subtly arched an eyebrow or asked an innocent question or showed me in any way that he did not understand or agree with my idea, I might change my mind.

Sue and I went for lunch, and I told her my idea. Thankfully, she strongly encouraged me to do it. And I did. About an hour before the time Brennan had been born the previous year, I drove to the hospital, six months pregnant with Kellan. My midwife, Nancy, happened to be on duty, and the ward wasn't too busy—both signs that this was meant to be. I asked if I could go into the room where Brennan had been born and lie on the bed. Nancy sat beside me and heard my plan, and then she left me alone. I needed to relive the experience and become close to him again on his birthday. With the staff's support, I did just that.

No balloons, no giggles, no cake, no family sharing his special day. Another dream lost. Instead, with my notebook and box of tissue beside me, I cried and cried as I tried to recall every detail. My arms ached again and I quickly used up the tissues. I wrote Brennan a poem and thought of the dreams that had been dashed when he died, and I said a prayer for all of the love and support David and I had received during the past year. I knew I was a different person because of his little life, and I found some gratefulness for my new mission of helping others in his name. After being back in my Grand Canyon of memories and grief, I pushed the button for Nancy as we had agreed. Together we talked of the upcoming birth of my next baby. We discussed plans and shared hopes and dreams for this baby, as well as the fear that something bad could happen again. Then after all of the emotional outpouring, I slept for about a half hour. Amazing! I had been so tense; it was shocking to realize that I had accomplished more than I set out to do. Brennan's day had evolved into a peace-filled nap. I could look forward to the next baby with some hope, not just fear.

After spending about two hours at the hospital, I drove to meet David as we had planned. We spent time in the place where we had scattered Brennan's ashes. It was a sweet, sad, and loving time. Then we went out to dinner. I am not sure that he felt as *full* as I did, since I had not invited him into my process at the hospital, but I doubted that he could have needed what I needed. He was very supportive of my visit there and assured me that he would have encouraged me to do it. I guess my own insecurities and uncertainties about it were being projected on him.

Almost one year after Brennan's birthday, I had my first-ever massage. As the therapist worked on me for a few minutes, she asked a simple yet powerful question: "Are you angry about something?"

I don't think of myself as an angry person and I knew for sure that during the previous year I had done everything I could to make good things come from bad—to help others, to feel better myself. In short, I strove to focus on the positive, which is a mantra of mine. But as soon as she uttered those words, tears poured out of my closed eyes and I couldn't speak for a few minutes. Then I realized that I had been holding boatloads of anger inside of me and hadn't even known it. The floodgates opened, and the massage therapist and I had a special chat about Brennan.

When I went home, for the first time I thought a lot about what I was angry about: everything about the way his loss was handled and the bad decisions we made, all the people who said, "It would be worse if he had lived for two years or twenty years and then died," and all that I was missing in our (what once seemed to be a "perfect") life. Mothering a mission could never come close to cuddling, rocking, feeding, nurturing, and showing love to a real, live baby. Yes, I was angry—but I didn't know what to do about it. So I wrote it down, I allowed it to live a little more openly in my heart. I named it and owned it, and then I moved on, because the mission called.

Just after Kellan was born, David phoned me one day. "I've never quite done anything like this before. I don't write poetry. But I wonder if you found anything on the desk, a poem actually. Why don't you read it and call me back?"

As I read the poem, tears flowed, and I understood that my loving, supportive husband, who rarely cried anymore and who looked to everyone around him to simply be a happy new father, still held his first son in his heart and lamented who and what was missing. Instead of the pages and pages and books that I wrote to express thoughts and feelings, he had done it in just a few words. His openness and willingness to share his vulnerable side with me brought us even closer together.

During subsequent years, we made many efforts to remember and include Brennan and our other babies in our lives. I made Christmas stockings and embroidered their names on them. We had birthday cakes, launched balloons, planted trees and flowers, included Brennan's name on greeting cards and so much more. Saying the names and sharing the love was sometimes an effort, but sometimes it felt very natural.

The manner in which I told Kellan (then three years old) and Trevor (then one) about their baby brother Brennan was another memorable moment. The boys were tugging at a sweet teddy bear that Kellan especially loved to play with. Kellan kept telling Trevor, "Give me my bear. It's not yours and I want it!" *Aha*! I thought to myself. *This is the moment I have been waiting for—a chance to tell both boys about their brother*.

My philosophy was that it was never too soon to tell them. So I sat down with them, gently took the bear and said, "Boys, I can see you both really like this bear. It is cute, isn't it? Kellan, I know that you have played with it a lot and think it is yours, but really, it is not. Before both of you were born, there was another baby born. His name is Brennan. Sadly, he died at birth and never came home with Daddy and me. This was his bear, given to him at a baby shower. He never played with it. But I am sure that if he were alive he would let you play with his bear sometimes."

The boys seemed mostly curious. Kellan (the verbal one at the time) asked a few questions, seemed satisfied, and then the boys moved on. Later that day Kellan asked what "that baby's name was." From then on, it was out in the open, and our Brennan conversations were rarely planned. I found other ways to explain the miscarriage of Marama and Bryna. My two living children seemed to accept that death was a part of life, which was one of my goals with my openness about our family losses.

In fact, when Trevor was five our neighbors, Tim and Barb, had a new baby. I told Trevor this and instantly he asked, "Mommy, did the baby live or did the baby die?"

I calmly answered, "He lived, Trev. His name is Tommy. But I understand why you ask that. You know that sometimes babies die, don't you?"

"Yes, like our baby Brennan." It was a sweet conversation, nothing morbid about it. I had hope that my sons would grow up and be able to talk about such things and face them squarely, unlike too many people I know.

When Brennan would have been five, David came home from work one night and suggested that we do something special for his birthday. I found that interesting, since the few previous birthdays had not seemed so significant to David, though they were for the boys and me. In the years since Brennan's birth, I have spoken with many, many fathers, and it has come out repeatedly that babies are not what most men dream of. Rather, fathers look forward to ages such as five when they can introduce their children to games of catch, fishing, wrestling, and so many other things that babies and even toddlers just can't do. David's need to be close to Brennan's five-year-old memory and find new ways to memorialize him then fit right in with these other men's experiences. So we found special ways to include Brennan and remember him on that birthday in November, and again when the bus came the first day of school the next fall. No little curly-haired Ilse boy would hesitantly or joyfully walk up those stairs on his way to kindergarten, but we could imagine him doing it, and the bittersweetness of it washed over us.

One time I recall when Trevor was five and Kellan was seven. We were in the car, and I reminded the boys that it was Brennan's birthday: he would be eight. Kellan began singing, "Happy birthday to you; Happy birthday to you. . . . You smell like a monkey, and you act like one, too." Trevor thought about this quietly for a few minutes and then said, "Kellan, don't talk about my baby brother that way." This caused quite a pause from his normally verbal older brother. A few minutes later, after rationalizing it all in his mind, Kellan said, "If Brennan were alive, he would be teasing me a lot, just like I tease you, Trevor. So that's why it's OK that I sing that song about him."

How to include our son in holidays was something we never quite figured out, but I did learn later of beautiful ways that other families did it. For almost twenty-five years I have shared how Kurt and Sue did it. They purchased a special candle after their little baby, Hope, died. They named it Hope's candle. Whenever either one had an especially sad or sensitive or emotionally charged time, he or she would light Hope's candle and the other partner would just know. This gave them a chance to connect and understand each other without words needing to be exchanged. On holidays, they carried Hope's candle with them to celebrations and dinners. Either on the table or counter, the lit candle stood as a reminder of their special baby who was not physically present, but present in their hearts.

As Kellan grew, he played with lots of kids who were one year older than him—children who would have probably been Brennan's friends. While I did notice that throughout the years that Kellan was growing up, the full impact of its significance didn't really hit me until it was the week before the high school graduation of what should have been Brennan's class. Kellan was really excited to go to the graduation, and actually a bit sad; some of his best friends would be leaving high school and he would miss them.

A day or two before the graduation ceremony, I revealed to David the scheme that was percolating in my head. I wanted to go to the high school graduation. "To prepare for next year and to see Kellan's friends graduate," I said to him. And in my head I added, *And to be close to my Brennan, creating more memories and imagining what it would have been like to hear his name called and watch him walk across the outdoor stage.*

The evening was as hot as a sauna, and as the not-yet-setting sun glared down on the metal bleachers, David's and my eyes locked with that *look*, and I instantly realized that I was not the only one remembering our baby and imagining him grown up and about to graduate. It was a special time we shared, as tears shed were hidden so those sitting next to us would not know. I think we explained it to Kellan and Trevor later, wanting them to also remember the significance of this day for the brother who lives only in our hearts and imaginations.

About a month before our dear Brennan would have been twenty-five years old, David once again surprised me. He quietly asked me what I thought about drafting a short piece to put in the memorial section of the *Minneapolis Star Tribune* newspaper. It was an unusual idea to me, something I don't think I would have suggested. Though I was always very open about our loss and the ensuing pain, I hadn't considered an ad in the obituaries after twenty-five years. Yet, the more we talked about it, the more the idea grew. I wrote a few rough drafts, and we agreed upon this.

Brennan William Ilse, Stillborn Nov. 2, 1981

25 years ago you came into our lives. No breath, no pictures, no footprints, yet you touched us deeply. You inspired an outpouring of love to others—through your story, *Empty Arms*, and more. You'll always be our son, our brother. Forever loved, always remembered.

Mom, Dad, Kellan, and Trevor

Then we sent this note to many friends, family, and care providers on the twenty-fifth anniversary of Brennan's birth/death:

Dear one and all,

Twenty-five years ago today, our son Brennan was born and had already died. As you know already, life changed dramatically and has never been the same. While many, many days, weeks, months, and even years were tough, there were also many gifts that have come our way. As David and I reflect on some memories, go off to visit the hospital where he was born and bear gifts, and go about our normal day, we are thinking of ALL the people who have touched us deeply, honored Brennan's memory, helped us in our journey to support and teach others, and who have just been (or become) our wonderful family and friends.

We are thinking of each of you today and hold a special place for you in our hearts. Thank you for everything, for being there, and for now being more sensitive to others in similar situations. Because of this, our mission, Brennan's short life, and YOU, the world is a bit of a better place. Thank you for allowing us to say in our own small way, *Brennan is forever loved and always remembered*, as it should be.

Hugs, blessings, and love to you.

All of this gave us a sense of satisfaction, for many reasons. We were publicly honoring and remembering our son who never even came home from the hospital, but was, and still is, deeply loved. We were thanking people who had been supportive and put up with my obsession—I mean, mission!—over all these years. And we were letting people know that a tiny baby can be loved and remembered for a very long time—in hopes it would give others the courage to hold their babies close to their own hearts forever.

I recently learned about the book *Final Gifts*, by Maggie Callahan and Patricia Kelley. In it, the authors collect and recount the last words of people in hospice programs. About one-third of the people about to die themselves spoke of little babies who had died, most many years before. This is amazing. And yet it is not.

Love cannot be measured by the size of a body or the length of a life lived. Rather, we love to the full capacity that we can love no matter how long we have had our children with us. The dreams and hopes that we parents have for our children begin early in our lives and may lie in our unconscious until we are physically expecting them, though we have long awaited them. The lifetime we have envisioned and built for our children and the love we cherish in anticipation of their arrival are real and significant. When a treasured baby dies too soon, and the dreams we hold in our hearts are dashed, there is one constant. And that is love. I am convinced that we can and should hold on to that love until our dying days. They, and we, deserve nothing less.

CHAPTER TWELVE

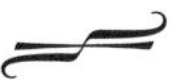

A Plan Gone Awry

Monica Murphy LeMoine

I wouldn't consider myself a lingerie-wearing type of person. Buying some expensive, impractical thing made of silk (that *has* to be dry cleaned, naturally) was not something that ever crossed my mind, especially not during my two-year string of pregnancy losses when my libido had all but evaporated. *Dead-baby mommas don't wear sexy, frivolous things! Nuh-uh no; we sit around in frumpy black attire and stare mournfully at the walls! Right?* That was my attitude, anyway. My poor husband, Kevin, went months and months without getting any action in bed.

I felt sorry for him, sort of.

Then one day as we were sipping our morning coffee at the kitchen table, he looked up from the newspaper sports section and said, "You know what I'd love? I'd love to come home from work one day and find you wearing sexy lingerie and scrubbing the kitchen floor." He took a swig of coffee and then added, "Or doing dishes."

I laughed uproariously, of course. We both did. What an absurdly antifeminist, caveman-like fantasy to have! Coming home to find your highly independent, reasonably intelligent, reproductively pathetic (and therefore deserving of sympathy), dead-baby factory of a wife doing something as subservient as scrubbing the floor? *In lingerie?*

"That's hilarious!" I said. End of conversation.

The next morning, though, I woke up strangely inspired to make a covert run to Victoria's Secret. I'd never been there, of course, but I knew it was situated somewhere in the bowels of the crowded shopping mall down the street. What would be the harm in skimming the sales racks, at the very least?

The timing was perfect, because this was to be the weekend of our monthly "urban getaway"—part of our mutual New Year's resolution to infuse our relationship with more post-dead-baby romance, whatever that meant. Each month, we would find a cheap Internet deal for a fancy-shmancy four-star hotel in our town, where we would spend one gluttonous night gorging ourselves on a sinfully vegetable-less, butter-bathed dinner at a French restaurant, drink lots of wine, stumble back to our hotel room, and then . . . well, you know the rest.

This month's getaway happened to coincide with Mother's Day, a time that—as we all know—is usually fraught with emotional peril for the millions of miscarriage-and-stillbirth "mommies" out there. "Mommies" like me, grappling with the surreal fact of having briefly been a mother in the scientific sense, yet with no real living child to show for it. And what better way to embrace my newly baby-less life than by boldly surprising Kevin with my first piece of real lingerie, waiting for him on our hotel bed in my slinky outfit as he stepped out of the shower?

I felt excited by the prospect—more energized than I'd felt in months. Years, maybe. So I told Kevin I was off to run some routine errands and drove to the mall instead, my heart going pitter-patter. Wandering into the perfume-scented Victoria's Secret with its sultry-eyed models gracing the walls, surrounded by strappy, lacy breast-cups and panties made of string, I felt oddly as though I were doing something illegal. Something that might land me in hell. Something my prune-faced fourth-grade teacher, Sister Estelle, would surely frown upon.

Old Sister Estelle would certainly have given me a hard whack with her ruler if she knew what naughty little number I soon found myself reluctantly and carefully slipping into, parading before a dressing room mirror. A tight black bustier that pushed my boobs upward with gravity-defying ease. Silky black garter belts clipped to thigh-high black stockings with lace around the top. Made in Italy. Perhaps a bit over the top, but I decided if I was going to do this, I might as well go all the way. And how remarkably human, feminine, *un-stillbirth-ish* I felt in this bold, skin-revealing costume!

After glancing at the price tag and swallowing hard, I decided to pay in cash. No need to leave a permanent record of how much I was about to pay for this black, silken ensemble—even considering the sale price.

That evening, Kevin and I set out for our usual, wine-infused French dinner. I was secretly wearing the bustier underneath my dress, minus the stockings. My carefully constructed plan was that later, while Kevin was taking a pre-bed shower, I would quickly yank the dress over my head, pull on the pantyhose, snap everything together (possible in ten seconds flat, the saleswoman assured me), and be lying in bed seductively when he emerged (not scrubbing the floor, but at least meeting *half* of his previously stated fantasy criteria). It was the perfect plan!

Well, almost perfect.

The dinner was, in fact, perfect. And the rest of the night would have been perfect too if, just as we were about to step into the elevator to whisk us back up to our room, we hadn't run head-on into the last bunch of people I expected to see. It was a giggling gaggle of ladies from the Seattle Urban Expecting Parents Meet-Up Group—the group of which I had been *the* original founder almost two years before. I had been the proud social queen of this group back in the day, head organizer of prego-lady parties and potlucks, all while carrying my doomed son Zachary.

Really, I only recognized one person: Cathy, the young woman who had stepped into my shoes as the group's new leader after Zachary was born dead. But I was sober enough to make a hasty educated guess that these were other, newer members who arrived later.

"*Cathy*?" I said. "Wow. Um, what . . . what are you all doing here?"

Her eyes met mine briefly before she gushed, "*Monica and Kevin*!" as her face lit up with recognition. She lunged forth to enclose me in a fierce sorority-girl hug, and then offered Kevin a quick cursory embrace before pulling away.

Kevin, who certainly recognized Cathy too (either that or was doing a damn good job of pretending), tossed his arm over my shoulder, pulling me ever so slightly closer to him. He knew as well as I did that the outcome of the evening—as with so many aspects of a stillbirth-couple's life—rested wholly on *my being* OK. It is, after all, the dead-baby momma who's left with the most lingering maternal sentiment, a fundamental fragility hidden deep beneath the walls of her strong and scarred heart. And this was precisely the sort of unexpected danger zone that could penetrate those layers of the heart, setting me off into an irreversible funk that might very well last for days. Not that I ever wanted to be the kind of person that slipped easily into funks—for *that* certainly wasn't the Monica that my husband had agreed to marry five years earlier. It was just one of those weird, subtle ways in which baby-death had taken hold of my mind over the years, transformed me.

With the side of my body against the curve of Kevin's, I suddenly felt the wiry seam of my naughty black under-attire pressing into my skin and remembered the exciting and sensual plans I'd dreamed up for tonight. I paid *money* for this body-hugging under-attire, real hard-earned money, and I was not going to let this little blip ruin my stealthily concocted plan!

Determined to keep emotion at bay, I flashed a brittle smile.

Cathy turned toward her friends. "Wait, let me introduce everyone. Guys, this is Monica, the one who started our group a few years ago! Remember I told you about her?" They all nodded and smiled, watching me. I felt myself inwardly recoiling as she spoke, memories of that former "me" flooding back like rapidly flipping pages of a cartoon booklet. Me, with my rapidly expanding belly. Me, a mother—sort of—or at least headed in that direction.

Cathy explained that they were all here for a little Mother's Day getaway—just a tradition they had started last year after all their babies had been born and they needed a mommy-getaway without the husbands and kids. So now every year they would get a group rate at the Westin, and . . .

Her voice trailed off as though she suddenly became aware of the meaning of her own words, of how they might feel and taste to me as they traversed the static air between us. How sharply they highlighted what could have been but never was, an imaginary future of parenthood, a new mother that I'd been achingly, joyfully ready to become for nearly eight months—but never did. A warm, moving ball of baby limbs and head and torso against my belly walls, gone hurtfully cold and still. An awkward silence settled over the conversation, random people zipping past and around us en route to the elevators, and she bit her lower lip as the conversation and the other women watched us both quizzically.

"So, Monica," said one of the other women, "your kid must be about our kids' age by now, right?"

Cathy turned positively white, her brow furrowing beneath the thick strand of dark hair that had fallen over her face.

"Oh, it didn't work out," I said, cocooning myself more tightly into Kevin's side. "But it's cool now. Anyway, have fun, ladies!"

With the merciful "ding" of the elevator arriving, Kevin and I waved and abruptly hightailed it out of there, pressing "12" for our floor, fumbling for the key card, not saying anything. Time felt blurry to my wine-coated brain, my throat dry, a dark and indefinable feeling pressing against my insides. Soon, we were back in our spacious room, sitting on the edge of the bed.

"You all right?" said Kevin, clutching my hand in his.

"What? Yeah, I'm fine. Just a weird coincidence, running into them here." As morose feelings of disappointment lapped at my insides, threatening to come up and out like bile, I remembered once more the silken bustier underneath my cotton dress, the black stockings and accoutrements wadded up secretly inside my backpack. *Hope*. A chance to embrace this new life of mine, as I'd been trying so hard to do. "Anyway, you should take your shower. I'm gonna see what's on TV."

Kevin nodded and disappeared into the bathroom. Meanwhile, I did everything just the way I had intended to, ignoring the dull, throbbing ache beginning to form behind my temples: pulled off my dress, slid into the stockings, snapped those gartery-strappy things in place, and positioned myself strategically on the bed. Diagonally and on my side, so that the full curve of my thigh and hip were in plain view.

But by the time the water shut off with a "thunk" and Kevin emerged with a towel around his waist, I was no longer lying seductively anywhere. Instead, I sat shriveled in a shadowy corner of the room, huddled on the carpeted floor. Like Cinderella missing the midnight deadline, I was no longer the sensual vixen I'd hoped to become tonight, but just my ordinary, crumpled, dead-baby-momma self. In a funk, again. Bawling my eyes out, getting snot on my brand-new lingerie, not caring.

Kevin sidled up next to me, not asking what was wrong because he knew. Men learn these things out of necessity as they walk along their own surreal baby-loss path, watching their women come apart and then get pieced back together in slightly different form, occasionally unraveling again. This was one of my unraveled moments, I suppose.

"I like you in that outfit," Kevin said after a while as I leaned against him.

"Thanks," I blubbered into his shoulder.

We sat like that for what felt like hours, eventually winding up under the covers and sleeping like an old married couple, not engaging in the rip-roaring sex I'd imagined. The next thing I knew, I was awake and squinting in the morning sunlight, standing in front of the mirror, still wearing my now-itchy and snot-crusted bustier. I felt dry and headachy and hung over, the taste of alcohol still lingering on my tongue. My throat was dry from breathing through my mouth all night, nasal passages clogged from my pre-bedtime sob session. I wondered fleetingly if I might have early symptoms of swine flu, but dismissed the idea before it had time to fester.

In the end, all was not lost. While Kevin slept in, I went for a stroll in the quiet downtown streets, guzzling Tylenol with water and infusing my bloodstream with several cups of strong coffee and a warm croissant. As my headache dissipated, I felt cleansed, refreshed. I hadn't enjoyed a good old-fashioned bawl-fest in a while, and—now that I thought about it—perhaps it was something I had needed. And besides, it was kind of nice that my lingerie was now christened with my own snot. Somehow it now felt more "mine" than it had in the Victoria's Secret dressing room, more blended with my stillbirth-mommy self than just last night. Feeling whole and caffeinated, I meandered back to our room, stripped down to my bare skin, slithered up next to my husband's warm body, and then . . . well, you know the rest.

Kevin remarked several times how much he liked the smokin' outfit. I told him that was fine and good, but not to hold his breath for the floor-scrubbing fantasy.

CHAPTER THIRTEEN

Saying "Grace": Family's and Friends' Responses to My Daughter's Stillbirth

Candy McVicar

"It is going to be perfect. . . . Our kids will grow up together and be the best of friends."

"They will be sweethearts and get married one day."

"You can watch the baby and it will be such an ideal setup for daycare, since our kids' ages are so similar and we live right next to each other."

"We can meet together at the park and have playdates."

"My husband will coach their sports team, and the boys will all play together."

"The timing is exactly how we wanted it; they will all be three years apart, which works so well with your kids' ages."

"We are going to have two sets of twins in the family now—how fun!"

"You are such an adorable mother and couple and you are going to have a gorgeous baby. . . . I can't wait to spoil her and dress her in the cutest outfits. She is going to have you guys—and all of us—wrapped around her little finger."

When I was a single woman and even married but without children, I attended so many baby showers and celebrations of friends as we eagerly awaited the arrival of the babes yet to enter our world by birth. I remember hearing the conversations; they conjured up imagery in my mind of things yet to come. The banter at times seemed like déjà vu—even though the circle of friends in each instance was altogether different, the conversations seemed all too similar.

There are natural expectations and norms within society when anticipating a birth and the ensuing days, months, and years for what will transpire in the mother's life and the life of the baby. Traditionally, there are celebrations, showers, ceremonies, and the like in the months leading up to and shortly after the birth. The mother is full of life and all things hopeful; she has many notions of how things will play out as this baby arrives and becomes the youngest family member.

All of these interactions and conversations had a profound effect over the years as they shaped my mind and the minds of these other women about what to expect as a mother. These words reverberate through my mind even now.

In May 2001, it was finally my turn. I had gotten married in my late twenties and was eager to start a family. My pregnancy let me enter the gates of this sacred and ancient rite of passage for a woman. All those tapes of conversations in my mind were playing out in my life as I got together with the different circles of friends and family. Both my sisters-in-law were pregnant, and six of my close girlfriends were expecting, too. There were four showers planned for my baby, and countless other baby showers for friends; it was a time of excitement and planning.

With fondness I remember the pictures on the wall of my mind. Sue getting on her knees and touching and kissing my belly, saying, "Can't wait to meet you—precious, dear little one." Having lunch with my girlfriends and sharing our dreams and excitement while downing the ice cream that we claimed was to satisfy our babies' cravings. Discussing labor and delivery with my girlfriends and being wide-eyed with wonder and fear as I pondered how I would handle labor. Would it go fast like it did for Sandy, who had her baby in the car on the way to the hospital, or would I break down and beg for all the pain medications when it dragged on too long, like others had shared it had for them? There were the stories of how some of the women passed a stool in labor on the birthing table and all of us listened, mortified at the thought. At the time it sounded like one of the worst things I could imagine happening during birth.

I left my corporate position to start a job I could do from home, and we began preparing for this little miracle to come into our lives. Once the worry of miscarriage had passed, my experience and knowledge up to that point in life told me that it should be fairly smooth sailing ahead. I had no idea about all the other pregnancy milestones, nor about how often things can go wrong along the way. My pregnancy was riddled with challenges, including severe hyperemesis gravidarum, the medical term for excessive vomiting, which I had for six months. Even with that difficulty, I remained very positive and excited about the baby's arrival. We decided to wait and find out the gender at birth.

I was due on Valentine's Day, but in December of 2001, I started noticing less and less movement. Some days I could hardly detect any movement at all. After two weeks of calling the clinic and going in for seven different visits to have Doppler checks to listen for the baby's heartbeat, I was finally given the ultrasound appointment that I wanted so badly. Finally I would get the chance to see what was going on and why the baby wasn't moving. I was concerned that the baby was sick or something wasn't right; though I was worried, I had no notion at all how severe the situation was. The ultrasound appointment ended up changing the course of our lives forever. To our shock and horror, we were told there was no heartbeat and our baby was dead. We were instructed to go to the hospital to deliver.

Anyone who has heard those words and learned that terrible news knows the unfathomable, heart-wrenching pain you feel at that moment, as well as the residual pain that continues for many months after. It is amazing that any of us, as stillbirth parents, is able to walk through and do what is required during those next hours and days. To labor, deliver, hold briefly, and say good-bye to your little baby who embodied a lifetime of hopes, dreams, and expectations and then simply hand over your loved baby to some stranger and walk away—it is a surreal and bizarre thing to live through. It feels like an out-of-body experience, as if watching someone else go through the motions, but not being in touch with how this is your own reality. Somehow we did it and we survived—it seems a small miracle that the experience alone didn't kill us. I think it was the shock that carried us through.

The grief that settled in like a bad cold in the chest that you can't get rid of, however, nearly took my life in the following months as I fell into despair, longing for my firstborn, Grace, who was no longer in my arms.

We were the only ones among our friends who had delivered a baby that was stillborn, so this was all new to us and to them. Our world had been turned upside down. What made sense before didn't make sense now.

Initially, there was a huge outpouring of support from friends, family, and even strangers all over the globe. The cards, care, and concern expressed were kind and sincere. However, the words spoken and written often left me reeling and caused me anger, hurt, and confusion. So many comments seemed more about comforting the giver than they were about comforting and helping us as the recipients.

"God doesn't give us more than we can handle."

"All things work together for the good."

"She is far better off in Heaven with the Father. He is taking good care of her."

"You will have more. There will be more babies."

"It must not have been meant to be."

"She was needed in Heaven more than she was needed here."

"Thanks be to God; He saved her from hell."

I would look at the person speaking with my jaw dropped and eyes wide. Usually quick with a comeback, I fell speechless, while many choice words filled my mind but found no way to exit my mouth. Had these people personally experienced having a stillborn baby, I doubt those stinging words would have ever passed their lips or even crossed their minds.

On New Year's, less than two weeks after Grace was born, my husband's family sat around our kitchen table having dinner. Only the sound of forks and knives on the plates echoed off the walls. The gargantuan elephant in the room was looming; no one seemed to have the ability to speak to us about Grace, so no one did. Though I tried, I was unable to sit with my two sisters-in-law, both of whom had huge pregnant bellies. I ran off to my bedroom to sob into a pillow. The pain was Grand Canyon deep; they had what I wanted, and my baby was gone while they got to keep theirs. The stories we had told each other about our children's lives together were destroyed, interrupted by the silence of Grace's birth. The family adventures and family pictures were forever changed now, and one little girl would always be missing from all those images.

As time went on, it became clear that our family was more comfortable moving on. No one else felt comfortable acknowledging her absence or our loss, so they avoided talking about Grace at all. Our communication and interaction became awkward and uncomfortable, and it stayed that way for many years. It is still heartbreaking to me when our families fail to acknowledge Grace's birthday. We send cards and gifts for each of our nephews and nieces, and if we were to forget even one, it would no doubt be brought to our attention and we would be reminded to send something. I have often thought about how it would feel on their end were we to bring to their attention all of Grace's birthdays they neglected, and how much that hurts. What if I were to say that we expected to see a card or gift in the mail soon?

Even though I know, intellectually, that families with stillborn babies often feel this kind of abandonment and loneliness after their babies are born, it still hurts. If only people without having lost a child could understand that the simple things said and done go a long way in bridging the gap often created in relationships because of the grief and loss. It really doesn't need to be much; a card that says, "We are remembering your precious daughter and we miss her too" would go a long way to making bereaved families feel love and remembrance of their babies.

In the months after Grace's death and birth, I learned how it really only takes one person in a group to make your grief worse, or to make it much better. My husband and I led a small group at our church for couples, and three of the gals had been pregnant when we were expecting Grace. All of them had their babies shortly before or after we had Grace. One couple had a baby with physical challenges who otherwise was healthy. The other two had healthy, happy newborns. Only one other couple in the group of six couples didn't have any living children. Though they hadn't been through any losses themselves, they reached out to us and offered support in considerate ways. We ended up hanging out with this one couple more than with the others because they helped us feel comfortable and safe and didn't offer platitudes. Also, the circumstances of our friendship made it easier to spend time around friends who didn't have children and who didn't talk constantly of what milestone their baby had just reached. We remain good friends with this couple even now.

But after Grace's birth, we started to distance ourselves from the other members and eventually ended up leaving the group. The new parents in the group felt hurt—they wanted to reach out and help us, not realizing that their way of helping was, at times, hurtful. They said things that stung our hearts. Their lack of exposure to stillbirth and lack of knowledge about the effects of grief prevented them from knowing what to say and how to help us. If asked today, I would venture to say that they learned a lot from watching us go through our grieving, and it now affects how they relate to others who are going through painful experiences. This is one small way—of many I have seen—that Grace's death was not in vain.

One of the most painful things was feeling as though others saw us as bad luck, angels of death, or pariahs. It seemed as though some people we knew saw stillbirth parents as carriers of a contagious disease, or bearers of bad luck. People avoided us and privately made decisions to exclude us from certain gatherings; this made me feel as though they thought our tragic situation would spread into their lives and create tragedy for them. In some ways, I can understand that we were walking reminders that bad things happen to good people. Pregnant friends learned what had happened to us and were forced to confront the fact that their babies' safety and well-being were not guaranteed. Our loss gave people a sense of how fragile life really is, and a stark notice that no one is immune to hardship. Unfortunately, many people chose to take the route of avoidance instead of facing that reality head-on and journeying with us through the valley. They wanted to remain as blissfully ignorant as possible.

This often left me—and me and my husband as a couple—to journey through that valley alone. If we brought up something about our grief when in the company of close friends, most would change the subject. If I spoke about my pregnancy when others were sharing pregnancy stories, the room fell quiet, and someone switched the topic. If a pregnant mom mentioned a concern for her baby, she'd remember my presence and then briskly move on, saying, "It's probably nothing." It was abundantly clear that no one wanted me to share or offer any suggestions.

I would walk away from those encounters feeling so angry and hurt. What if one of them had a stillborn baby? Would they look back at when they ignored the lessons I could have shared from my baby's situation? Or would I bear some responsibility or sense of guilt because I had kept my mouth shut and not said something that could have helped save their baby's life?

As uncomfortable as my pregnant friends felt around me and my baby girl's death, I felt similar discomfort around their big bellies. I was jealous and I longed for what they had. Even worse was being around those mothers who had foul attitudes during their pregnancies, who complained about their babies and their living children.

I wanted to hit them over their heads and say, "Wake up! Are you blind? How can you be saying these things? Don't you realize the gift that you have? Start appreciating this baby and be grateful."

I also looked at women who had full bellies and prayed a quiet prayer that their babies didn't have to die. But at the same time, in the very same prayer, I conversed with God about why they got to have their babies and we didn't.

While the world goes on and babies are born all around us, often there are few who show lasting compassion for those who have lost a baby. It is very challenging to turn from our sorrow in order to celebrate with joy for others. And it's a gift of mercy when a person can grasp that we are on a long and difficult journey, and can compassionately offer enduring patience and kindnesses to help us through.

There are those with whom I, thankfully, do not have to put on the mask of being OK. Friends who have joined me on the path of grief understand when I just say, "This sucks," and they know firsthand what a "bad" day or week means. There is a peace I feel when I am among others who can really relate to my experience and appreciate fully the feelings that "outsiders" from this club cannot comprehend.

And there are the new words and conversations that heal my heart and nurture loving memories of my daughter.

"I miss Grace. I wish she were here with us. She would have been an amazing little girl and we missed out," I cried.

With tears flowing down her face and a kindred heart of understanding, her own heart after also having suffered a painful loss, a friend listened as I openly grieved and simply said, "I know. I know, sweetie. It hurts so badly. It's not going to hurt like this forever, but for now, let those tears flow. Grace is worth every one of them."

Others I've gotten to know through our organization, Missing GRACE, have spoken words of healing and comfort, too.

"Grace is one very special girl with one very incredible mom. . . . You are a great mom to Grace, and I believe she is very proud of her momma."

"I am thankful for all you do for Grace. You have helped me and countless others and your work is an inspiration that has made me want to do more and to find ways to remember my baby."

CHAPTER FOURTEEN

Our Christmas Angel

Laura Villmer

Christmas for me was always a time for family and a time for celebrating the birth of a baby. When I was a child, my cousins and siblings and aunts and uncles would crowd together on my grandparents' front porch and sing "Happy Birthday" to Jesus as someone placed the baby figure into the nativity scene.

Now, my Christmas holidays are also about the death of a baby. My husband and I and our two little girls huddle around a pink headstone and sing "Happy Birthday" to our angel, as one of us puts flowers in the vase and one of us tries to light candles.

Our second daughter, Madeline Lucille Villmer, was born still on December 25, 2004. I was 35 weeks pregnant, due in late January.

That holiday season was supposed to go like any other. Go to see the in-laws for dinner and presents, attend Mass at 11 p.m., and then wake up Christmas morning to watch Hannah, our twenty-one-month-old, find her presents from Santa Claus. We were planning on celebrating Christmas with my family on December 26.

Charlie and I were both twenty-seven, and we had been married for four years. This, my second pregnancy, while unplanned, was definitely not unwanted. Even Hannah was excited for Baby Madeline's arrival.

We woke up on Christmas Eve to no electricity. No electricity for us also meant no water, so we grabbed some toiletries and clothes and drove to my sister's house to clean up and hang out for a little bit. As I sat on the couch relaxing, my mom put her hand on my belly like she always did and asked how Madeline was doing today.

Her question made me stop and think. As hectic as the morning had been, I hadn't paid any attention to the movements in my abdomen. After 35 weeks (and with this being my second pregnancy), the movements were just happening. They were just another part of a pregnant woman's life.

"Actually, she's been really quiet," I said.

I told myself that surely she had moved, and I'd just been so busy that I hadn't noticed it. I went on with my day.

We went home for a little bit, and then drove to celebrate Christmas with Charlie's dad and his family. At first I kept my fears to myself; deep down, I think I knew something was wrong with Madeline, but I didn't want to think too much about the possibility that something was truly wrong.

So I sat at the kitchen table chowing on chocolates and drinking sweet tea, trying to get a good sugar rush to the baby to get her to move. Nothing. I reclined in a chair and played a game on my Palm Pilot; she'd always kick me where my hand pressed into my belly, but not that night.

After a bit, I told everyone that I didn't think I'd felt Madeline move all day. They tried to reassure me, saying that she was probably just sleeping and that babies usually move less at the end of a pregnancy. Yeah, I'd heard that, too. Sure, she was just sleeping. That had to be the reason why I hadn't felt her moving like normal. There couldn't be something wrong with my baby.

We exchanged gifts with Charlie's family—I got a cute little baby outfit that, it turned out, Madeline would never wear—and we went home. I got dressed to go to Mass in one of my favorite maternity outfits: a black and white polka-dot shirt and black pants. My stomach was upset, and I felt slightly nauseous. I thought it must have been the chocolate I had gorged myself on.

But when I got into the church and knelt down to pray, I found myself praying to God to make her move. *Save my baby. Do something!* The hour just dragged on and still no movement. I tried to focus all of my attention on my baby bulge, holding my hands still on the sides of my belly, trying to feel any slight movement. I didn't sing as much as I normally would and didn't pay too much attention to the Mass. My mind was elsewhere. *What would happen if something truly was wrong? What would we do?*

I went home and tried to sleep but couldn't. Charlie went through box after box in our spare bedroom until he found an old stethoscope he had from when he worked at a hospital. He moved it around tenderly on my belly and said he thought he heard two heartbeats. I couldn't even hear my own heartbeat with it, so it was no good to me.

I finally gave in at about 2 a.m. and called the doctor's emergency line. He called me back quickly and said, "We'll get you in and hook you up to the ultrasound, and you'll be home in time for Christmas dinner."

Still trying to convince myself that nothing was wrong, I called my mom and asked her to drive me to the hospital while Charlie stayed home with Hannah, who was sound asleep.

At the hospital, a nurse hooked me up to the fetal heart monitor but couldn't find anything. After several minutes, she tried another monitor. Still nothing. So another nurse came in and tried, too. By this time, I was in a flat-out panic. My mind was trying to convince my heart that something was wrong, but my heart kept arguing back. *Maybe they had faulty monitors.* But two of them? *Well, maybe she's just hiding really well in there.* But surely they'd find some trace of a heartbeat.

The nurses called in my doctor, and he brought the ultrasound machine with him—the machine that would show me that my daughter was still alive but just sleeping peacefully, right?

Wrong. The ultrasound confirmed my worst fears. My daughter, whom we'd seen on several ultrasounds during the pregnancy alive and kicking, lay there motionless. The little heart that we had seen so many times before thumping and beating furiously now was silent.

I lost it. I held my mom and cried, and she cried, too. Everyone else left the room, leaving us to our grief.

I made my mom call Charlie, because I just couldn't tell him that our daughter was dead. I still wish that he had been there with me instead, and that we'd heard the news together.

Charlie dropped Hannah off at my sister's house and drove to the hospital. My mom started making phone calls to my sisters and family members and friends. It was about 6 a.m. I started to feel some uncomfortable cramping—labor was beginning. Our doctor told us that we could go home and celebrate our Christmas and come back in a day or two to deliver the baby. That thought was slightly morbid to me: walking around with a dead baby inside me, acting as if nothing had happened. Worse yet was the thought of having to answer everyone when they asked me why I was crying uncontrollably.

No, we decided, we wouldn't wait. We chose to go ahead and deliver, so they hooked me up to the pitocin drip and gave me an epidural. My original plan for labor didn't include an epidural, which made me feel like even more of a failure.

Family members started showing up. My dad. All three of my sisters. My brother. People called to tell me how sorry they were. My grandma, with whom I am very close, called from vacation in Texas to ask if I wanted her to come home. I told her no, there was nothing she could do for me except pray. She had suffered miscarriages before and knew what it was to lose a baby.

And now, the only grandbaby to be named after her (they share Lucille as a middle name) was gone. I found myself feeling sorry for my grandma.

Everyone else had Christmas plans that day. My older sister and her husband took Hannah with them and let her open some of their presents with his family. We kept her totally oblivious to the tragedy. We didn't see the need in telling her about it, when she couldn't fully comprehend.

And sitting there laboring painlessly, I realized that we'd have to plan for after the birth. I'll never forget the look in Charlie's eyes when I told him that we'd have to bury our baby. He sat at the foot of my hospital bed with his head hanging, but once I reminded him of the funeral, he raised his head and looked at me. His eyes held everything I felt: fear, shock, disappointment, bewilderment, and pain. That look still haunts me.

Thankfully, my parents took care of all of the planning and all of the phone calls. I lay numb in the hospital bed, trying to convince myself that it was all a dream. In reality, Madeline was still alive. She'd be born crying and pink just like her older sister was.

But again, all of my attempts at convincing myself couldn't change reality. Madeline was born still at 1:20 p.m. in a cold, sterile, and eerily quiet hospital room. There were no cries of joy and no wailing baby. No oohs and aahs from the nurses. Just silence.

They took Madeline at once to the corner of the room and cleaned her up. Then they brought her to me so I could hold her.

I made the most of that time, trying desperately to memorize her face and her smell. I stared at her face, hoping to imprint the image on my brain so that I could never forget. I knew that my time with her was so short. I passed her to Charlie, who cried just as I did. Then my mom and dad came in and held her, too. We pulled her little hat off to look at her hair, and unwrapped her blanket to check out her toes, too. She had a full head of black hair, just like her older sister, and long skinny fingernails that already needed clipping.

She was perfect.

I'm not sure how long I held her, but I knew that I couldn't hold her forever. As much as I wanted to never let her go, I knew that I had to give her up. I can still feel her cool skin on my lips as I kissed her forehead for the last time.

My mom had asked if I wanted her to take pictures, but the hospital staff had said they'd take one, so I told her no. That is my worst regret. The only picture I have of Madeline was taken hours after her birth, and she's not the same perfect little angel I remember so well. I wish we had pictures of her being loved, being snuggled in our arms.

I was given a room at the end of the maternity hallway, far away from the happy parents and their babies. More people came to visit and more people called. It was a relief not having to be alone.

We were released the next day after giving a hospital employee the information for the death certificate. Instead of Charlie wheeling me out while I held our newborn baby in my arms, we walked out together, hand in hand.

As we stood waiting for an elevator, a proud new father wheeled out a mother and baby. They waited for the elevator's arrival. I pulled Charlie back; I couldn't ride on that elevator and inhale all of that cheerfulness when I felt none of it.

I was surprised by how hard it was to leave the hospital. It felt like I was leaving her behind. But I knew she wasn't there, even in body, anymore.

My family had been planning to celebrate Christmas on December 26 that year, so we went ahead with the gift-opening tradition. I spent most of that day watching Hannah—I couldn't take my eyes off her. I held her as much as I could. I played with her hair and just watched her as she opened her gifts and played with her cousins and laughed.

It was difficult to be around so much joy after such an emotional ordeal. I was there, but I felt vacant. My eyes were tired from crying so much and from lack of sleep, and I really did not want to be around so many people. I faked happiness and probably even laughed a little bit, but I felt hollow.

And we still had to live through the funeral. We opted for just a small graveside service. The thought of standing in a funeral home while our friends and family came by to offer condolences just didn't sit well with me. I didn't want their pity, and I didn't want them to feel awkward as they tried to come up with something to say.

We got the burial plot next to my mom's parents—I wanted Madeline to be with family in heaven.

On December 29, we made the first walk up the hill to Madeline's grave. I was worried about Hannah. What would she think or do during the service? But I saw out of the corner of my eye that someone was getting her out of the car as we got out, and I focused on Madeline again.

Our chairs were placed on top of my grandma's grave, and I silently asked her to hold me up and give me strength.

I don't remember what was said at the funeral service. I felt Charlie's hand in mine and could hear his sobs, too. I felt my dad's strong hand on my shoulder, and I wished that I hadn't sat on the end of the line of chairs. I wanted to be sandwiched between my husband and my mom, to feel as much love and support as I could.

After the service I was stunned by all of the family and friends who were there. The hugs just kept coming. My immediate family, of course, and Charlie's family, and our closest friends were there. But then there were aunts and uncles, coworkers (my office had closed that morning for the funeral), and old friends from grade school and high school. They all came out to give us their support, and we needed it.

I found Hannah after the service, still sleeping in her Uncle Bryan's arms, oblivious to her parents' pain. And we tried to keep it that way. We told ourselves that we couldn't break down and cry all day long. We couldn't lie on the couch in a grief-stricken stupor and ignore the needs of the child we still kept with us.

I found a new determination to be an even better parent, and a better me. To focus more of my time on the child still sleeping silently in the room down the hall, instead of crying and agonizing over the one sleeping in heaven.

I really felt like I had no choice but to keep going with my life. I grieved, and still do, over my lost baby and her lost life. The future we never had with her. The incomplete family pictures on the wall.

A little more than a year later, we got pregnant again. Extra precautions were taken during the pregnancy and delivery, and our nerves were shot, but Clara Leigh Anne was born in September, happy and healthy as could be. And our world became a little bit brighter.

The pain of losing a child will never go away. I feel my tears well up at random times. Sometimes, the sadness is connected to Madeline in an obvious way—when I watch my nephew Jaxon, who was born just two weeks after Madeline, hit various milestones in his life, or when Hannah drew a family picture in her preschool class and included Madeline. Other times, I'm caught off guard by emotion—like the first funeral I attended after she died, and I was surprised that I had such a hard time leaving. It brought me right back to Madeline's funeral, when the thought of leaving her, yet again, overwhelmed me.

And of course, Christmas is always a time of joy and pain for us. Just when we think it might be getting easier, we realize it never will.

We've tried to incorporate Madeline into as many of our Christmas traditions as we can. She still has a stocking, and it hangs on the wall with all of ours. We keep it empty, because there's really no gift we could give her. We buy an angel-shaped ornament for her every year, and make a point of hanging the "Baby's 1st Christmas" ornament that my mom had gotten her that fateful year—appropriately, an empty cradle—on the tree first.

We take an angel off our church's Giving Tree each year and buy for a child in need. We've never been lucky enough to get a child who would be Madeline's age, but we still want to buy for that child as we would have bought for Madeline.

My Uncle Fran recently gave us a beautiful cabinet to display all of the angels and things we got at Madeline's funeral. It sits in our living room for everyone to see.

My sister, Cindy, drew Madeline's picture for us, since we don't display the picture from the hospital. Cindy's drawing hangs in a prominent spot in our house.

Every Christmas, as I watch my daughters opening presents and join my family in the next card game, I mentally relive those two days from 2004. I remember what I was doing and how I felt, building up to the moment of Madeline's birth.

And then we get in the car and go to the graveyard to sing "Happy Birthday" to Madeline, our precious Christmas angel.

Having Madeline's birthday on Christmas is both a blessing and a curse. I love that the day she blessed us with her presence is not some random day, some day that everyone else will forget as the years go on. But then, I find it hard to feel as happy as I used to on Christmas. I have to carve out my personal time to really grieve on Christmas Day, which usually is about the time when we visit her grave. It's a difficult balance—being happy and sharing the holiday joy of two daughters, while mourning the daughter who never will share in that joy.

Hannah now knows all about her little sister, and she talks about her frequently. Clara, at the moment, is a bit young to understand. But, when the time comes, we'll tell her about her older sister who spent just 35 weeks here on this earth and who is now her personal guardian angel, watching over her and making everything all right.

During all of my pregnancies, I always felt as if I was in on some "inside" joke, talking and laughing in my head with my tiny babies. I always felt like there was someone with me constantly, as if I were never alone.

And now, I know I never will be.

CHAPTER FIFTEEN

She Was Significant

Nina Bennett

I fell in love with my grandchild the moment my son, Tim, called to tell me I was going to be a grandmother. His older brother has two children, so I was well aware of the pure joy of grandparenting. Tim's wife, Jenn, had a glowing, healthy, full-term pregnancy. A vegetarian, she was vigilant about nutrition. She and Tim had researched birth options and chose a holistic medical practice staffed by nurse-midwives. Tim and Jenn had a carefully thought-out birth plan. They wanted their baby born in an atmosphere of love and tranquility. I had taught childbirth classes for many years and was extremely involved in the natural childbirth movement, so I was quite pleased with their choices regarding prenatal care and delivery. Tim and Jenn did not want grandparents present during labor and delivery; they planned to call us when their baby was born, and we would join them to greet and toast our newest family member. When they called to tell me Jenn was in labor, I went to work. My digital camera and cell phone were in my briefcase, batteries fully charged.

Tim called me frequently throughout the day to give me updates on Jenn's progress. Toward the end of my work day he told me that Jenn was six centimeters dilated. The hospital where I work is mere blocks from the birthing center where they were delivering. I live about thirty minutes south of the city. I knew that by the time I drove home, Tim would call me and I would then need to turn around and drive right back—both trips made in rush-hour traffic on the turnpike. I am not an assertive person and my son had expressly stated that they did not want grandparents with them, yet in a statement that is totally out of character for me, I told Tim that I was coming over to sit in the waiting room. I assured him that I knew I would not be with them. His response was also uncharacteristic—without trying to talk me out of my decision, he said, "OK."

My entire life changed a few hours later when Tim stood before me in the waiting room and without making eye contact said in a monotone, "I need you to come upstairs. We had a baby girl. She doesn't have a heartbeat." I hurried up the steps after my son, questions tumbling out, the nurse who accompanied him saying gently, "We've called neonatal transport; we don't know what happened."

The scene I walked into was a nightmare I had never once contemplated. The entire staff was frantically working on my granddaughter, performing CPR and attempting to start her heart with medication. I went into autopilot mode and retreated from my role as a grandmother to my professional training and experience as a health care provider, for to acknowledge the horror of what was taking place was more than I was capable of. I knew how to be a professional assisting a family in crisis; I had no idea how to be part of that family. The neonatal transport team arrived and took over the CPR and resuscitation effort. The birthing suite, intended to be a welcoming setting of serenity and joy, had deteriorated into controlled chaos and barely concealed panic. The soft music chosen to accompany my grandchild's entrance into the world had been turned off, replaced with terse medical orders. Finally, after an excruciating forty minutes, the doctor called off CPR, and Madeline Elise was officially pronounced stillborn.

I was numb. The entire situation was surreal. We held Maddy for hours. I carried her around and talked to her, singing lullabies, telling her how much I love her, memorizing her features and the feel of her in my arms, basically cramming a lifetime of grandmothering into a finite amount of time. I drove home that night, feeling more alone than ever before, pulling into my driveway with no recollection of how I arrived there. I lay down on my bed fully dressed, dreading the coming dawn, not knowing how to face a life without my granddaughter.

The next morning I nervously took the memory card from my digital camera and downloaded the pictures of Maddy. Because I was crying and shaking as I took them, I expected the pictures to be blurry and out of focus. I tried to mentally prepare myself as I opened the file on my computer. When I viewed them, I was astonished; every single picture was in perfect focus. I sobbed as I gazed at Maddy's perfect, beautiful features. This could not have happened. There was no way that this pregnancy, so wanted, so healthy, so well attended, could have ended in death. Her face in those pictures is completely serene; it is obvious there was no fetal distress.

The following days passed in a fog. Each morning I got out of bed certain that Maddy's stillbirth hadn't really happened, that today Jenn would go into labor and everything would turn out fine. Flowers and meals arrived constantly. I begged my parents and my oldest son and his family to come over to eat. I thought it ironic that the standard thing to do when there has been a death is send food, yet I had absolutely no appetite. My phone rang nonstop, but I didn't want to talk to anybody. I moved through the days in slow motion, as though I were standing in a shadow watching myself. I am not a good sleeper to begin with, but after Maddy's death, I had terrifying flashbacks of CPR being performed on Maddy every time I started to drift off. I heard the plaintive tone in my son's voice as he begged the staff to assure him that his daughter would be OK. Tim's anguished wail when he opened the car door the night his baby died and saw the carefully installed infant seat reverberated through me. I tried to use distraction therapy with myself and replace those scenes with Maddy's peaceful face as I held her. I wasn't able to cry when other people were around, and I really preferred to be alone. I couldn't bear to hear any sound, even the voices of family and close friends. I felt removed from their conversations—voices heard across a vast chasm, sounding as if they were underwater.

With my granddaughter's stillbirth, I became a member of a club nobody wants to join. A club whose membership fee is astronomical, yet once joined, you are a permanent member. A club defined not by gender, ethnicity, religion, profession, or political beliefs, but by a single immutable fact—the death of a child. A club whose membership pin isn't proudly displayed on a collar or lapel, for the jagged pieces of a broken heart aren't readily visible. In the days after Maddy was born still, I searched desperately for validation of my grief. The raw, wrenching pain I felt was like no other I had ever known. I had no familiar context in which to place my loss. I felt isolated by an experience nobody wanted to talk about. I longed to speak with someone who didn't flinch at the word "died," who didn't turn away in horror and pity at the word "stillbirth," who knew better than to offer empty platitudes. Life continued on around me in a blur, but nobody seemed to have any concept of the depth of my pain.

Corporate policy on bereavement leave is a prime example of society's ability to overlook the reality of a grandparent's grief; standard time off granted for the death of a grandchild is one day. When I returned to work, not one person asked me my granddaughter's name or weight. People did acknowledge my loss, but nobody validated Maddy's life. Friends and coworkers kindly asked how my son and daughter-in-law were coping; rarely did anybody ask how I was doing. I did, however, receive many commands on how I had to be strong for my son.

I must admit that I resented every single time somebody voiced that. I didn't feel strong. I didn't want to be strong. I wanted to sob. I wanted to scream. I wanted desperately for somebody to tell me that it was OK if I did. I actually needed to be given permission to grieve.

I lost not only the hopes and dreams that accompany a new baby, but also the joyful radiance of my beloved son. Tim, always a private individual, completely withdrew from me. To witness the pain and heartache of my child, the bereaved parent, was unbearable. As a mother, I was used to fixing the problems my children faced as they grew. When my son was learning to walk, I could pick him back up if he fell down, give him a hug, and tell him he was OK. When he tumbled off his bike, I could clean his cuts and scrapes, put a big old Spider-Man Band-Aid on, and make it all better. During his teen years, I could advocate for him and advise him after a traffic ticket that in a few years the points would come off his record and it would all be forgotten. Now, I was finally confronted with something I couldn't fix. Not only was I unable to fix it, I couldn't even make it better. I have never felt more powerless. I cried as often and as hard for my son as I did for myself. I couldn't even think about how my son must be feeling. Knowing the intensity of my pain, contemplation of the depth of his pain was unimaginable.

At first, I was consumed with the very process of grieving. I felt as though I was engaged in a monumental battle of endurance, with grief being a formidable enemy. I was devastated by the loss of my granddaughter, distraught at my inability to soothe the pain of my son and daughter-in-law, and hurt by a society that did not want to acknowledge a grandmother mourning a stillborn baby. I completely reject the often-used terms *resolution* and *closure*, as they simply do not exist for me. To speak of closure implies that we get over the loss and move on. To resolve, to let go, to move on, means denying my family history. Not only does this diminish Maddy, it diminishes my sense of who I am and my place in the world.

Instead, I am concentrating on redefining normal as it pertains to my life. So much about my life and who I am changed with my granddaughter's stillbirth. To say that the experience of losing a grandchild has made me a better person is too simplistic. Although I have been profoundly changed by the stillbirth of my granddaughter, in many ways the change is more of a transformation. Some of these changes have indeed been positive, such as a commitment to living my beliefs about the importance of family. The values that I formed during the sixties, such as actively appreciating the beauty around me rather than taking it for granted, have been strengthened. Much of my innocence about life, however, has been shattered. Time has taken on new meaning for me. I no longer believe in tomorrow. My inner sense of security has been shaken, and I am more tentative about relationships. I find it very difficult to take anybody's continued love or support for granted. Some friendships have fallen by the wayside due to a lack of understanding and acceptance of my grief. However, the friendships that weathered the unpredictable storm of my grief have become richer and fuller. I tend to be more withdrawn in social situations, and I lose interest in casual conversations quickly. I've always been introspective, and while I am by no means a loner, I find that I need more quiet time than ever before.

I am a bereaved grandmother. This is the defining element of the new normal that is my life since Maddy was born still. I am reminded on a daily basis of how precious each moment is. I make time to nurture meaningful relationships. I consciously work at placing my family first. I am committed to being fully engaged in living life joyfully, for to do less would dishonor my living grandchildren as well as Maddy. My grief journey is integrated into my life journey. Maddy leads me every step of the way, showing me that life is indeed beautiful and worth living. I pay particular attention to the moment just before day slips into evening, when the colors in the sky deepen until they seem to slide off the horizon. I am astonished by the brilliance of the stars. Did they always sparkle this brightly, or is the effect enhanced when seen through the prism of my tears? My tears may lessen over time, but they will never dry up, nor will they be forgotten.

Maddy has taught me a vital life lesson—the ultimate beauty is found not in the destination of the journey, but in the scenery along the way. When I see a dragonfly, my family's symbol for Maddy, I know Maddy is reminding me to slow down and appreciate my surroundings. What an amazing legacy left by a baby who never drew a breath. My heart will always contain the joy, excitement, and love I felt for the nine months of Maddy's existence. She is part of me, child of my child; I will forever be her grandmother. As I sat through Maddy's memorial service, the funeral director repeatedly spoke the phrase, "She was significant." It was as though he wrenched those words from my heart and seared them into my brain. I am determined and absolutely committed to perpetuating Maddy's legacy through my writing and public speaking. I will not let my granddaughter be defined solely by the stark fact of her death.

I am slowly learning to make peace with grief, for I understand that it will be with me always. I realize that grief cannot be outrun. By turning and facing it head on, I can own my grief, rather than have it own me. I savor every sunrise and sunset, and I pause often to gaze up at the stars. On a clear, crisp winter night, when the sky is as dark and heavy as velvet, I feel a gentle snowflake brush my cheek and imagine that Maddy is blowing me kisses.

CHAPTER SIXTEEN

How Death Can Bring Life: A Caregiver's Perspective

Kathleen Skipper

As a labor and delivery nurse for many years, I have held families in my arms both through joy and through sorrow. And my heart has been touched in both instances. I spent over forty years learning and teaching about perinatal loss and the effect these kinds of losses have on parents, families, and health care professionals. It certainly is not an easy topic, but it is one that must continue to be pursued until there are no more babies who die.

My most profound teacher about perinatal loss was my firstborn child. I had always dreamed of becoming a mother. Becoming a labor and delivery nurse only fueled this desire. After five years of marriage and many tests for infertility, our dream finally came true . . . I was pregnant! We were so thankful and overjoyed.

My pregnancy passed uneventfully until I was in my ninth month. I reached 41 weeks' gestation and there were no signs of labor. Because of my irregular menstrual cycles the doctor felt we could have miscalculated my due date. So the days ticked by until my 44th week. My membranes ruptured; before we left for the hospital a great foreboding overtook me. I was experienced in checking fetal position by doing Leopold's Maneuvers, an external examination to determine fetal position. The doctor had told me the baby was breech, but I was feeling a large body mass on the top. How could this be my baby's head? The part I was feeling was soft and large, not hard and mobile.

When we arrived at the hospital I was taken to X-ray to have a pelvimetry done; this is an X-ray of the size of the baby versus the size of the pelvis. The doctor was there with me, and I asked him if the baby's head was all right. He replied that everything would be fine.

The obstetrician left me and went to tell my husband that our baby was not breech and that he had a condition known as anencephaly (absence of the brain). He suggested to my husband that I not be told until after I delivered.

Throughout my thirty-six-hour labor, my husband supported me with calmness and love. He would take breaks outside the room and cry. There was no one there to support him, to hug him, or to comfort him. He would dry his tears and come back to be by my side. This went on hour after hour, until finally I was taken alone to the delivery room. My husband was left to wonder and worry about what was happening to me and our baby. He had no idea if the baby would be born alive or not. All he knew was that our baby's condition was not compatible with life. If he wasn't stillborn, he was certain to die within a few hours of being born. What must he have gone through in those horrendous hours all by himself? Avoidance by the staff was more than obvious, and that has stuck with my husband to the present moment.

I was given a general anesthetic, so I was unaware when our baby was born. I remember nothing of the delivery itself. When I awoke in the recovery room, the doctor was at my side compassionately holding my hand and saying, "I am sorry. Your baby was born with anencephaly and will not live long." I asked him the sex of the baby, and he said, "You delivered a little boy." I was stunned. Shock and numbness immediately took over. Jim came in to be with me, and we just cried. The doctor told us that it would be better if we didn't view him because of his condition. It would be better if we just went home and tried to make another baby. So we agreed not to see the baby. After all, the doctor knows best! In hindsight, that was the worst decision we could ever have made. This decision haunted me like a thief in the night for many years. My subconscious struggled to answer the horrifying question: "What kind of mother could let her baby die in a nursery all alone with his parents in the next room?"

The well-meaning physician advised my husband not to talk to me about our son, whom we named James Patrick. It was seven years before Jim talked to me about his experience, before I learned what he had lived through the day Jimmy was born. We were on a Marriage Encounter and had three more children by then. I had a silent, dark emptiness in my heart that I tried to bury alive. Because grief has no timetable or set of months or years to complete, hearing my husband talk about that day for the first time took me right back to the moment of our loss. As Jim shared his story with me, all I could feel was an immense love for him and a great deal of guilt that I had put him through all this. Guilt was a weight I carried on my shoulders about everything! Discovering Jim's perspective on losing Jimmy just added to my feelings of guilt. I didn't know that guilt was part of the normal process of grief that I had been avoiding.

Immediately after Jimmy's death, his body needed to be buried. I was still in the hospital, and I was not permitted to attend the burial. Actually, no one even told me he was being buried. It was decided *for* me that it would just be too painful. It seems everyone was trying to protect me from my heartbreak.

Later, I learned that my husband carried Jimmy's little white casket to the open grave. Jim was accompanied by my father, his father, and a cousin, Jerry, who was a Catholic priest. Our son was placed in Jerry's family plot; no marker was allowed to grace his grave. I have only a crucifix that adorned his casket as a reminder of our son. I am so grateful for that cross now, as a reminder of my God who knew my suffering.

Twenty-eight years after Jimmy's death, I accompanied a young family to the burial of their stillborn daughter, Olivia. When Olivia's daddy carried her little white casket to her gravesite, I was suddenly whisked back in time, and it was Jim carrying our son's little casket to be buried. It was on that day that I finally buried Jimmy. It was a tremendously healing day for me. I will never forget Olivia or her beautiful parents, or the gift they gave me in being able to lay my son to rest.

Another comfort was that, against the advice of many others, Jim and I named our baby boy. That brought some peace because in my mind I knew I had a baby boy and his name was James and I still loved him.

In the postpartum unit, James's life was not acknowledged as a profound loss, but as something that happens with great frequency. I was given no assistance with my grief or comfort for my aching body. One nurse, however, gave me some unsolicited advice: "Stop crying! You are not the first woman to lose a baby, and you won't be the last!" Those words seared themselves into my subconscious. The only good that came from having those words hurled at me was that I promised myself right then that, as a nurse, I would never say anything like that to a bereaved parent. I have kept that promise, and I have also come to realize what some nurses must go through before they understand what a loss like this means to a family.

Not all of the nurses were callous about my son's death. One labor and delivery nurse told me how beautiful my son was, and that his body and face were perfect. That stayed with me, and her kindness comforted me often during the early days of my grief.

Two unexpected people who visited me while I was recovering in the hospital provided great comfort to me as I reeled with grief over James's death.

One was a Jesuit priest, Robert Burns, SJ, who was president of Canisius Jesuit High School, where my husband taught. He pulled a chair next to my bed, sat down beside me, and took my hand. Tears poured forth from his eyes, and he was speechless. I was touched to the core by his empathy. The other was a Sister of Mercy, Sister Jean Baptiste, whom I had worked for at Mercy Hospital. She spoke the words, "I am so sorry." I will never forget those two people and the grace with which they supported me.

When I came home from the hospital, my loving mother-in-law had cleaned out the room that was to be the nursery. With no crib or layette, it looked as if there was never any hope that a tiny infant occupant would come live with us. That ripped at my heart, and I struggled to understand why I didn't feel appreciation for her efforts. I know she was trying to help, but I felt so angry. I wanted to scream at her! On top of anger, I felt guilt for feeling so angry. But I squashed those feelings, burying them deep within me.

At times it felt as if I were going crazy. People advised me to behave in ways that didn't sound like what my heart was telling me at all. They told me to forget; all I wanted to do was remember. They told me I was lucky Jimmy died because I could have been burdened with a retarded son; I would have taken him any way I could. They told me to get pregnant again and replace the baby who died; I didn't believe I could replace him. I didn't want to replace him. They would not talk to me about the baby; all I wanted to do was talk. I wanted to visit his grave and no one would take me. When my husband went to work, I would sneak over to the section of the graveyard where I knew Jimmy was buried, and I would just sob and sob. There was no one to talk to . . . no one to listen to my broken heart . . . no one to help me embrace the naturalness of my pain. I was a woman of faith, so I talked to God, screaming, "Why me?" Confronted with the loneliness and sadness, I had to work hard to believe I wasn't crazy for having all these feelings.

I went through physical, emotional, psychological, and spiritual pain that I had no idea how to process. I entered a dark hole and buried my pain alive for nearly thirty years.

I didn't know it in the days and weeks after Jimmy's death, but I have learned that what is buried alive stays alive until you can embrace the pain and embrace your grief. When I neglected the lifelong presence of grief over my baby's death, I thought I was successful in getting over it. But the mind and heart have a way of bringing that buried topic to the surface again. My memory of those days is like a tape recorder: just push the button and it all comes back as if it were yesterday!

Jimmy's short life and death have touched more lives than I could ever have imagined. Before he was born, I loved being an obstetrical nurse, but I never could have foreseen the places where Jimmy's life would take me, and how his death would help not only bereaved patients, but also many health care professionals. I believe that Jimmy's life was a gift not only to me but also to hundreds of families that I have had the privilege to assist through the beauty and pain of pregnancy and infant loss.

In my career as a labor and delivery nurse, I was acutely aware of what the death of a baby meant. I had endured it. In the late 1960s I began, on my own, suggesting that parents view their stillborn babies. As I lovingly held their stillborn baby, the parents would often ask to hold the baby themselves! I know now that, when they saw that I wasn't afraid of death, of their baby, or of their pain, it imbued them with the courage to extend their arms and hold their babies themselves. Of course, the tears flowed. But as I had promised years before, I did not try to stanch the tears. Instead, I realized that my actions, far from bringing more pain to the bereaved, were actually acknowledging the pain that was the natural outcome of love and hopes and dreams.

I began receiving letters of gratitude from all the parents who saw, held, and touched their stillborn baby. The parents whose babies had been stillborn or died soon after birth were expressing their gratitude far more than the parents whose babies had been born healthy. This was incredibly significant, because I started to realize, through my actions with other babies and families, that my own son's death was overshadowed by the ways I was not allowed to grieve him. Throughout the 1970s and 1980s, I observed parents in this horrendous and unasked-for position. Yet somehow, the support and encouragement I was able to provide to others was healing me. I was doing for them what I had missed so deeply.

Early on, nurses and doctors couldn't understand how I could encourage families to enter into such pain. I even had some doctors accuse me of causing the parents more grief. But even though many people disagreed with my actions, no one stopped me. I even shared with the physicians and nurses that my biggest regret was not having seen or held my own baby who had died. I told them I felt if I had seen my son, my healing would have been more possible.

Before long, I conceived of the idea of taking photos of these beloved babies who had died too soon. I brought my own Polaroid camera to work and took pictures of stillborn babies—with the parents' permission, of course. Then my peers *really* thought I was going off the deep end! What good could come from taking a photograph of a baby's corpse? Even though others were horrified, there's no doubt in my mind that Jimmy was leading me.

I continued doing these so-called outlandish things and wrote down what I observed. I just intuitively knew that these things—encouraging parents to see and hold their baby, offering photos, and supporting parents through the postpartum grief process—were the right things to do. Through the 1970s and into the mid-1980s, I had no written information that what I was doing was supportable in any research. Then in the late 1980s, I received some literature from a program called *Resolve through Sharing*, a training program for health care professionals and others who were interested in helping those going through the loss of a baby through stillbirth or newborn loss. I couldn't believe my eyes! Now there was a program that had been researched and established. There was literature supporting my theory. I wasn't just some crazy nurse driving newly bereaved parents off the edge. Reading the supporting brochure, I was out of my mind with peace and joy.

In the meantime, the OB unit where I worked was closed. Soon, I was hired at a larger teaching hospital. I grieved the closing of the small unit where I had worked, and I balked at going to a much larger unit. But there was another plan I couldn't see. The head nurse at the new facility had heard of my interest and expertise in providing support after stillbirths and newborn loss. She approached me to ask if I would establish a program. The hospital even sent me to *Resolve through Sharing* for training and coordinator training. Formal training in what I had already been doing was a gift of affirmation; it made me even more determined to share with others what I had observed and experienced.

I felt as if I had a mountain to climb, to help others in the health professions take a new approach to helping newly bereaved parents. I took one step at a time, letting things unfold naturally. First, I gave educational seminars to the nurses on labor and delivery. Some got it right away. Many didn't; some resisted because it's destabilizing to be presented with something that runs contrary to our educational beliefs. The new way required coming out of their "safe places" and really getting engaged with the dead baby's family. Many of the nurses felt like it was risky to step outside of the box. Some nurses expressed a fear of facing another person's pain. They would exclaim, "Oh, I couldn't do that! It is too painful!" But as they came to realize that it wasn't about their pain but rather the pain of the patient, they saw the loss from a different perspective.

Before going to work, I prayed for courage to continue to be a patient advocate. Being at the forefront of this change in my area was sometimes a very lonely spot. Swimming against the current, I was led by my heart and by well-researched material. Slowly but surely, the seed that I was planting took root.

Many of the nurses and doctors bought into the ideas I presented. Far from just sharing my own experience in working with patients, I provided documented literature. I distributed checklists for all health professionals who come into contact with patients. I mentored those who were interested. Nurses who had never experienced a pregnancy or infant loss themselves were transformed into absolutely wonderful supports to our patients. The first year of the program, I started Caring Arms Support Group, a group primarily for parents who have had a stillborn baby. The attendance was astounding. We started a memorial fund to provide the financial support for the program. A memorial garden was constructed on the grounds of the hospital. More support groups developed: miscarriage, interrupted pregnancy, family and grandparent, and subsequent pregnancy groups were added as the needs presented themselves.

We held our first Walk to Remember in 1991 with sixty-four in attendance. In 2010, there were more than five hundred who came. From a tiny seed grew a mammoth tree!

Other nurses and some doctors, social workers, and pastoral care personnel traveled to attend our training programs. We held annual conferences, and we continued to find that the more education people received about grief and infant loss, the better the care our patients received. Doctors gradually began to see the usefulness of the program and bought in to its concepts. They realized that, instead of parents leaving their practices after losing a baby, most patients returned if their physician had supported them.

Unfortunately, even to this day many health care professionals would like to avoid discussing stillbirth, perinatal death, and all that those kinds of losses entail. As someone who is both a health professional and a bereaved parent, I have come to believe that these doctors and nurses are not necessarily mean or cold-hearted. Rather, they are *afraid*. Some are afraid of death. Some are afraid of their own emotions. Some are afraid of their humanity and their inability to fix this kind of pain for their patients. Some are afraid that the brutal pain of losing a baby or child could happen in their own families. Some are afraid of saying the wrong thing. How can you deal with the unimaginable? Doctors often take the death of a child as their own personal and professional failure. And unfortunately, some physicians and nurses who don't want to learn more about these losses avoid their patients' pain completely.

In medical training, we are taught to cut out the diseased part, bandage the wound, and take away the pain. That is why it is such a contradiction to learn that it is sometimes necessary to help patients embrace their pain, that this process of feeling the pain instead of assuaging it can actually bring healing. Added to the ideological and philosophical challenges doctors face in learning how to help patients cope with pregnancy and infant loss is the fact that physicians are pressed for time. It takes time to sit with a patient, to listen to her, to walk up and down with her on the journey of grief. It's not billable to the insurance company. Doctors may feel more comfortable prescribing an antidepressant to solve the problem. While there are certainly cases in which antidepressants can provide much-needed support, this approach can sometimes erect a Plexiglas wall over the doorway through grief on the way to healing.

Though much progress has been made over the past decades since my Jimmy's birth and death, the education must continue. The death of babies is never an easy issue to address. Parents whose babies have died are wonderful educators and advocates. But the most important quality necessary for moving forward is the commitment of people to share their stories, people to listen, and communities to support patients through the difficult work of grieving. Through this process, not only the patients are helped—the health care professionals enter a realm of healing and love that brings new life to them, giving them a greater capacity to care for those around them.

From my perspective, parents are the best educators. They need to praise doctors and hospital workers for the care they provided, or write to express disappointment when care was lacking or insufficient. Parents can contact hospital administrators to educate them about the ways in which good support programs work. Where there is no program, show them the need to establish one. Our babies who have died are not without the power to help us make necessary changes. Hospitals want their patients to leave satisfied with the care they received. Thus, bereaved parents must write these administrators to give them input about the support offered for coping with the loss of a baby.

As a former nurse and coordinator of a bereavement program, I believe that the death of a baby need not end there. We may not be able to carry forth the myriad dreams we had for our baby, but we can help make a difference for others. I am so grateful for my son, Jimmy. He taught me so much.

He taught me the needs of bereaved parents.

He taught me that love never dies.

He taught me the importance of creating memories.

He taught me the importance of facing my pain, embracing it, and going through the doorway of grief.

He taught me that I have a chance of becoming either bitter or better.

In time, I have learned that his life was not in vain. His short life led me to help others embrace their pain and come to learn more about themselves.

All the bereaved families who have crossed my path have enriched my life. Through allowing me to walk with them, they have helped me grow in faith and love. Jimmy has brought me to new life, and I believe that all babies who have died have a gift to give. You only need open your hearts to all the possibilities that are out there. Your babies have great possibilities; they only need you to go forth and give their lives meaning.

CHAPTER SEVENTEEN

Invincible No More: What My Daughter's Stillbirth Taught Me about Life

Tim Nelson

At approximately 12 noon on September 27, 1983, life as I knew it stopped. After receiving an anxious phone call from my wife, Monica, telling me that something appeared to be wrong with the baby we were expecting any day, I drove to the hospital, totally unaware of what was happening around me. It was as though the world had paused in silence, and I was the only one still moving. The defining moment that phone call represented was followed by a quick succession of more of the same: when the doctor reviewing the ultrasound screen turned to us and said, "I'm sorry, there is no sign of life"; when only hours after those words were spoken the first flowers of condolence arrived in our hospital room; and finally, when our daughter was born into a world she would never see.

The silence of those early moments quickly gave way to chaos, and along with the turmoil came a sense that the life I thought I commanded was spinning wildly out of control. What I didn't realize at the time was that it would be months before some semblance of order returned and I would once again be able to "hear the music." Even then, there was the horrific realization that the universe seemed to be playing a different tune—one I had never heard before and was totally unprepared to dance to.

I was in my late twenties when Kathleen, our second child, was born still. Up until that point in my life I had, for the most part, viewed myself as someone who could accomplish nearly anything I set out to do. I thought that with hard work and a strong belief in myself, there was little I could not achieve. But like many people who experience a devastating event in life, I began to define my existence in two parts—before her death and after. There was much more clarity for me in understanding how my views about nearly everything I valued changed after her birth. Things that had at one time seemed important no longer were. Relationships with friends and family were altered; I measured them by how supportive I felt those people were of our circumstances. In addition, some of my naïve viewpoints about life evaporated before my eyes—like the belief I clung to that as long as I worked hard and was a good person, nothing exceptionally horrible would ever happen to my family or me.

Shortly after graduating from college I married Monica, the woman I had started dating when I was seventeen, and we quickly settled in to the task of starting our careers. She began working as a nursing home social worker and I launched a publishing business with a college friend. Monica and I had talked since high school about our desire to eventually have a family, but we wanted to spend time gaining financial stability as well as enjoying married life together before taking that step.

After three years of marriage we decided it was time to start having children. The first indication that we were not entirely in charge of our future presented itself when Monica was unable to get pregnant. But following many months of fertility testing and frustrating visits to the doctor, we found out that we were expecting twins. The roller-coaster ride continued when, six weeks after that good news, we learned during an ultrasound that one of the fetuses was not viable and we were at risk of losing both babies.

In the end, Monica gave birth to a healthy little girl we named Emily. And I convinced myself that the scary time of uncertainty was a mere hiccup in my otherwise calm existence. I once again began to believe we were indeed on track to live the American dream.

It was almost two years to the day after Emily's birth that Kathleen died. As our world seemed to shatter around us, both Monica and I drew on the resources we had accumulated over our lifetimes as a way to cope and keep moving forward. For Monica, her strong Catholic upbringing provided her with a faith that gave her a sense of peace and acceptance to which I had trouble relating. Monica also benefited from the close relationships she had with her fifteen siblings; they showed emotion easily and naturally, and she found strength not only in that support, but also from what she had learned facing adversity during her own childhood.

Growing up in rural Minnesota as part of an exceptionally large family resulted in Monica's forging special bonds with her siblings that many people never experience. There was a lot of love to be shared, and the entire family practiced the wisdom of enjoying the simpler things in life. But there were also unique challenges that accompanied her circumstances. At an early age, Monica acquired the ability to be strong and fend for herself. She was the eleventh child with five younger brothers, so she learned to not only stand up for her own needs but also support others with theirs.

When Monica was in her early teens, her parents began to struggle with alcoholism. Through that difficult circumstance, Monica gained further independence and an understanding that there were things in life that she could not control. Additionally, the family moved frequently during Monica's adolescence, so she learned to adapt to changing situations; she also gained an appreciation for the fact that her siblings were her one constant source of support.

I, on the other hand, had not really ever had to deal with anything that left me feeling so completely helpless as when Kathleen died. My childhood had not been perfect, yet nothing had prepared me to understand that there would be times in life when I would so clearly lack command of my destiny.

My only brother was three years older than I was, and he was a high achiever. As kids we had very different interests and goals; he was the straight-A student who was extremely focused on his future and excelled at nearly everything he tried, and I was the more social and less serious one. Circumstances never dictated that either of us depend on the other for more than the rather mundane day-to-day needs that siblings share in growing up. I considered myself lucky then, and still do, but the stability I appreciated reinforced my belief that only hard work and commitment were required to take me nearly any place I wanted to go, and that nothing could stand in my way if I wanted it badly enough. Even though I had to work harder than my brother to achieve different things, I nevertheless saw myself as the captain who steered my life's ship to avoid the icebergs.

The constancy of my family life clearly gave me a strong sense of who I was and a belief that my parents would be there to help and guide me in any way they could. At the same time, my family was not physically or verbally demonstrative. The love we felt for one another was real, but it was not spoken. While I certainly did not feel that presented a major obstacle for me at the time, I cannot deny that as an adult I found it very difficult to show emotion or openly display affection in public. I had come to believe, through my own interpretation of life events, that to seek comfort or cry in front of family and friends—much less strangers—was a sign of weakness. Over the course of my life, I had slowly and unknowingly built a protective emotional wall around myself. When Kathleen died, that wall stood between me and everyone else—including Monica.

The most difficult part wasn't that I could not understand the need to reach out to others, but instead my inability to know *how* to do that. I was simply incapable of letting my guard down, and as a result I sought ways to avoid situations that would put me in positions where I might be at risk of letting that happen.

In the early hours after being told that our baby was dead, I looked for ways to have the nightmare end as quickly as possible.

After hearing the ultrasound results, I vehemently resisted when Monica wanted to go home for a period of time before doctors induced labor. I wanted everything to begin immediately. Not only did I want it all to be over, I knew that leaving the hospital would put me at risk of coming face to face with family members or friends. The likelihood of my breaking down and losing control of my exterior emotions terrified me.

When the nurses at the hospital later explained what was apt to occur both during and after the delivery of our child, I panicked at the thought of someone offering to let me hold our baby. I wasn't nearly as afraid of our baby's dead body as I was of the possibility that I would shatter into tiny pieces and lose control over my emotions at that moment. When we were told that we could spend as much time as we wanted with the baby after the birth, my angst only grew more intense.

The hospital staff also suggested that we encourage family members to come to the hospital and see the baby, as well as take pictures. I drew the line at that notion and simply said no. I felt threatened by how I would act if that were to occur, and I wanted to protect my parents from the discomfort I (wrongly) thought they would feel if asked to come. Monica did not share my views, but between being in a state of shock herself and realizing I was near the edge of what I could handle, she went along with my decisions.

Certainly there were many instances during those early hours where I sought to manage situations I felt threatened my protective barrier. Those same defense mechanisms persisted in the months of grieving that followed, such as when I fought the idea of attending a support group or talking about my sadness with Monica.

My anxiety even extended to the first anniversary of Kathleen's birth. Monica wanted to spend the day together: attending church, going to the memorial stone, and having a little party so Emily could sing happy birthday to her sister. I was mortified at the thought that I would not be able to hold it together during the Mass. In addition, I still carried some anger toward God for letting Kathleen die. In short, the idea of spending the day remembering the hellish nightmare we had lived a year earlier depressed me beyond description. Adding to my anxiety was the fact that Monica had gotten pregnant again only three months after Kathleen was born, so we were expecting a baby any day. I had spent nine months refusing to let myself get excited about the baby's birth, and remembering the day Kathleen died only reminded me of all I had to fear—and lose.

Luckily, I had learned something about myself during that year of grieving. I slowly started to recognize that I could not rely on my initial instincts in situations that jeopardized cracking my emotional shell. I had come to trust that Monica's judgment was often better than mine at times like that. I subdued my fears and we spent the day exactly as she wished.

I was astonished that it ended up being a beautiful day, filled with far more happiness than sadness.

There is no doubt that Kathleen's birth and death forced me to reevaluate a great deal about my perspective on life and the realities I face as a human being. The most significant realization I made happened over time, little by little: that exposing my naked fears would not destroy me or my relationship with Monica. There is no better example of that than the lesson I learned the night of Kathleen's birth. As much as I tried to control the details of what occurred during those dark hours, some things were unavoidable. I simply could not escape the dreadful silence the moment she was born, or the undeniable stillness of her body when she was handed to me wrapped in a little white blanket. In the end, no amount of strength or level of reasoning could effectively counter my overwhelming sadness, and for the first time in twelve years of knowing Monica, I sobbed uncontrollably.

As I learned that showing emotion was an acceptable personality trait, I also gained a greater level of compassion for those experiencing difficulty in their own lives. I discovered that even though it is futile to search for magic answers as a way of comforting a person who is grieving, there indeed is something magical about a sincere hug and willingness to listen.

I would never maintain that only one event, even one as traumatic as the death of our daughter, is solely responsible for the growth that I have achieved over the course of my lifetime. However, a great deal of what defines me as a person today was altered by that event.

When I finally was able to recognize that my intense drive to always remain in control was the very thing most hampering my ability to grieve, I began a slow reevaluation of my outlook on life. That search for answers continues today. While I still believe I hold the key that can unlock my future happiness, I am endlessly reminded that I am powerless over some events. Whether it be finding myself helplessly standing by as a bad economy threatens my financial future, or waking up to discover that depression has silently crept into my being and is eroding my self-confidence like a cancer, I can no longer pretend to be immune from life's challenges.

With the aid of professional guidance and a tireless self-examination, I continually seek to make the distinction between the battles I command and those I must surrender. There is no doubt that Kathleen's death was the first major attack on my quest for complete happiness. But with the help of time and hard work, I can now see that the love she brought into my life was worth the casualties my ego endured.

CHAPTER EIGHTEEN

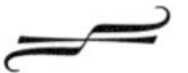

Reunion Group

Amy L. Abbey

We are the group graduates, the parents who have survived our nightmares. There are a handful of us these days, although our silent numbers reach into the hundreds here on Long Island, and thousands across the world. We are the ones who can journey back to those macabre days in an instant, the ones who can recall taking the steps on our journey in even more detail with the passing years. The further along we are, the more details we can procure—as if in each telling some new morsel of information, long forgotten, comes to light.

It is a crisp autumn night. I walk into the basement at the end of a long hallway, to a room I have come to know well. The small room is stark, as are its furnishings. It is unevenly lit, a chalkboard hanging on one wall, a bank of tables on the opposite one; the chairs are positioned in a semicircle, half in the light and half in a delicate darkness. I wonder whether the chairs were deliberately set this way or if they were haphazardly placed. The door is ajar. This one little room feels cold and uninviting. Entering, I feel great sadness and trepidation.

Inside the Pediatric Conference Room, I see one familiar face. It is the face of someone I have known for years, someone I would never have met had my life turned out as I had planned. Anna.

Though it may sound clichéd, Anna was my savior, the person who rescued me from danger and harm. Anna was my group leader and therapist after I lost Solomon. I smile and walk hurriedly across the room. Taking off my coat, I smile at the others gathered: three women and one man. They all seem calm and collected. I don't recognize any of them, so I assume these are the "newbies," the ones who will benefit from my story and leave knowing they will live another day. They are all grouped together on one side of the circle. So far, I am the only one here from my team.

As more people fill the room, Anna and I chat. She asks how I am, how Eric is, and how my kids are. My youngest child recently had a hospital stay for some undetermined illness, which brought back my intense anxiety and fears of loss. Now, I confide to Anna that if something had happened to Adam, I would have placed Solomon's picture with him in the coffin. It is a morbid thought, and I know that women who have not gone through my ordeal would never think this. I wonder myself sometimes how the story of Solomon can be so far from my daily mind, then spring to the forefront, jack-in-the-box-like.

Finally I see some familiar faces and feel relieved; I am not alone. That is always the point to remember. Sadly, there are others. I smile at Jeanine, Joey, Linda, and Diana. I am glad to see them all, and then it occurs to me: I am the senior "reunioner" here.

These loss group programs run throughout the year in six-week sessions to help the newly bereaved work through some of their grief. The meeting tonight is the reunion group, where former group members come and share their stories to help those who have recently experienced a pregnancy loss, ranging from miscarriage to stillbirth, to see that life goes on even after the tragedy of a baby's death.

Anna is joined by another social worker, Margaret; the two women introduce themselves and start the group's meeting. I can feel my heart start to race, knowing I will soon be introduced and asked to speak. My mind runs through the memories of what I will share and I take a deep breath, preparing to speak and hoping my voice doesn't crack. And then, as if the room darkens and a spotlight shines, I am on.

"Hello. I am Amy Abbey. I lost my son Solomon on March 8, 2000."

I pause and breathe deeply, feeling the lid rising off the pot of my sorrow. "At 19½ weeks pregnant, my water broke. I remember it clearly. It was a night like so many others. I fell asleep watching television with my husband, but I was awakened by a feeling of wetness and realized immediately that something was wrong.

"Eric drove us to the hospital in complete silence. We passed the mall where, just the day before, I had purchased my first maternity item, a bra. At the hospital I was ushered into the emergency room. I remember sitting in the middle of a row of plastic attached chairs, next to my husband. I sat clutching my copy of *What to Expect While You're Expecting* as if it were a

Bible. I wanted to check in at Labor and Delivery, but hospital policy or maybe New York State law forbade it. I was not pregnant enough; I had not reached that magical 20-week mark.

"I was triaged by a nurse and taken to an examining room. The resident came in, his name long forgotten (I wonder if I ever knew it), and examined me. The look. The look he gave was knowing and utterly honest; he looked grieved by the situation he must have known we would face. My situation was grave and he was not at liberty to discuss it with me. I was hooked up for an ultrasound and saw my little guy swimming inside—or was he bouncing off the walls of my uterus, since so much of my amniotic fluid was gone? I couldn't tell, but I was hopeful for a happy ending.

"By this time, my OB had arrived. Wearing glasses and a windbreaker, a departure from his usual professional doctor clothes and contacts, he didn't resemble the man I had come to know over the years as a gynecologist. His presence was reassuring as we prepared for a long night.

"I was admitted to Potter 2, the general gyn floor of the hospital, at about 3:00 in the morning. My bed was on the door side of the room, another patient on the window side. I would learn that this woman had had twins earlier that day. At this point, I believed something would be done to maintain this pregnancy.

"The next morning, I had another ultrasound. This time, the technologist would not let me see the screen. I knew the baby was still alive because I could feel movement. There was conversation by the staff about 'pockets' and 'fluid' and other things I tried to understand.

"After the ultrasound, I was wheeled back to my room, but complained to the nurse that I had heard they might be moving me. I was hopeful it would be to a treatment place in the hospital so that I could wait out the healing my body needed so that I could carry my baby to term.

"Sure enough, before I entered the room with the twins-mommy, I was taken to a new room on another side of the ward. I didn't know a black line had been placed on the door hanger outside my door so the staff would know something was going on.

"When my doctor came in, he told my husband and me that my amniotic fluid was gone, and since it was a complete break of the amniotic sac, we needed to do what was best to maintain my fertility for future pregnancies. He said because I was so early in my pregnancy, the best plan would be to induce me.

"Even now I try to recall what I was thinking, and I just come up blank. I didn't know you could induce someone so early in a pregnancy, or what would happen to the baby. From that point forward, I asked every intern or nurse who entered my room what the baby's chance of survival was. All told me the same thing: he probably wouldn't survive.

"On Monday evening, I started getting suppositories to begin labor. The evening news was running a segment on maternity fashions. I could not believe the irony and turned the television off. Around 3:30 p.m. on Wednesday, I delivered my baby into the silence of my room, with only my husband and my doctor present. My OB told me to push. I thought he was crazy. If I pushed out the baby, I could no longer hold on to the fantasy that this wasn't happening. I knew the baby had died, but the moment he was pushed from my body, that was it—there was no going back to the fantasy. Ever.

"Margaret came to see me before I was discharged," I said, smiling at her across the room. "To this day, I don't remember if I had seen her earlier than this. She gave me some pamphlets and telephone numbers to call if I needed help. I took two weeks off from work, and was actually home for a week and a half.

"I had promised myself that I would put this behind me, when I left the hospital empty-armed and broken-hearted. But by the second day at home I couldn't take it. I called and left a message on Anna's answering machine. When she returned my call, I specifically said I would come to a support group but that I didn't know if I would stay. I did not want to sit in a room with other crying women for two hours; I just couldn't see the point. I had never hated talking to another person on the telephone as much as I hated that conversation.

"But when I actually came to group, what happened was life-transforming for me. I met other moms like me: teary-eyed, angry, questioning. We shared our stories, we cried, we were silent, and we connected. Group was so much more than crying; it was about finding a new normal, a way to grieve our loss and integrate it into our lives.

"I learned through the help of Anna and Margaret that the baby I had delivered was a boy. I named him Solomon, which means 'peace.' I also experienced hemorrhaging for the entire postpartum period, and at seven weeks after Solomon's birth, it was so massive I had to have a D & C. To my horror I had to miss a group session and just felt so *wronged*. Then a week later, my OB suspected I had deep-vein thrombosis. While in another hospital emergency room, I told the doctor if he didn't discharge me to go to group I would walk out AMO—against medical orders. Eric assured him that I wasn't bluffing. Luckily, the pain wasn't actually caused by blood clots, but even if it had been, I would have left to go to group.

"When the six-week group session ended, I had new friends.

"My husband and I were finally given the green light to try again. It took four months before we found ourselves pregnant again. Still very much grieving for Solomon, I professed to Anna in a private therapy session that I would not have this baby. She assured me this was a common thought experienced by moms who had lost pregnancies. But it turned out I was right. The pregnancy officially ended on October 23, with another D & C, this time for a blighted ovum.

"I was seeing Anna about monthly at this time. My husband and I were supposed to wait to try to get pregnant, but I was insane and waiting was just not an option. I never thought I would be one of those women who took their basal body temperature daily and made love based on when we were most likely to conceive. But tragedy changes us, and I found myself keeping a handwritten temperature chart and maintaining one online. We got pregnant when we weren't supposed to, waiting only one cycle after my second D & C.

"Since no cause for losing Solomon was ever identified, my OB suspected my premature labor might have been caused by incompetent cervix. So, 14 weeks into my third pregnancy, I had a cerclage placed and began taking vaginal antibiotics for the remainder of the pregnancy.

"I was in denial most of those nine months. I saw Anna privately about once a month, always denying I was having a baby. It must have seemed ridiculous because I was huge and wearing maternity clothes. Anyone looking at me would have had no doubt I was having a baby. I allowed myself to enjoy my baby shower and for those three hours felt like a normal person—and I have the pictures to prove that I looked and acted like one, too. But every other moment of the pregnancy, I was overwhelmed by fear. Even after I had passed my loss-point with Solomon, I continued to feel my anxiety increase instead of decrease.

"The day before I gave birth I had an appointment for a nonstress test at my OB's office. I told him I was just about at the end of my rope. He implied that if I called the office in the morning and complained that the baby wasn't moving as much he would deliver me the next day.

"At 9:05 a.m., Tuesday morning, August 14, I called that office as fast as my fingers could dial. I told the nurse I felt a little off, like maybe the baby wasn't moving as much. I was now 38 weeks. An hour later I had an appointment in the operating room for later that afternoon. It was not here at Winthrop, but at a different hospital. I admit I was scared because delivering at Winthrop was part of my plan.

"On the drive to the hospital, I was crying. Eric tried to be reassuring, but I just could not listen to his happy-talk. I believed this would just be another trip we'd take to the hospital, only to come home empty-handed.

"Alison Rachel was born August 14, 2001, screaming her head off. It was the most beautiful sound I had ever heard. I felt the grief physically leave me, an albatross removed from around my neck. I fell in love with her immediately.

"When Alison was eleven months old, my husband and I found ourselves pregnant again. This pregnancy started slowly; my hormone levels weren't rising as expected, and I spent a few weeks in a panic. But things started to progress and everything was uneventful until I went into preterm labor at six months. Those contractions really hurt but not as much as the emotional upset that another pregnancy might be lost.

"I was rushed to Labor and Delivery and hooked up to the monitors, but by then the contractions had stopped. I was sent home. After another round of contractions a few days later, my doctor put me on medication to stop them and he put me on house arrest. I was only allowed out to go to doctor's appointments and Subsequent Pregnancy After Loss Support Group (SPALS).

"I desperately needed the SPALS group—I had gleaned so much support and encouragement from a SPALS website from the time I lost Solomon until months after I delivered Alison. But while the website helped immensely, I wanted a real human connection, in person. So during this pregnancy, a SPALS group was offered at Winthrop. One of the wonderful women I bonded with, Patty, became a great friend.

"Adam was delivered, happy and healthy, on March 28. Patty had Margaret track me down at a different hospital to make sure I had gotten my happy ending. It was one of the greatest feelings in my life, to have a friend who 'got it' so fully."

At this point Anna jumps in and asks me to tell the group what I am doing now.

"I published a book," I begin again, excited to share.

"From the day I came home from Winthrop after losing Solomon, I journaled. I wrote down my feelings about the loss, the grief, how I was feeling, how people were treating me, and the unfairness of my life. When I was pregnant again, then again and then again, the frequency of my writing lessened, but the emotions and thoughts were constantly at the forefront of my mind.

"Once Adam was born, I realized I could not take care of two children under two and write a book—I wasn't a writer. In my former life I was a health educator. What made me think I could write a book?

"That's when I decided to ask others to work with me. I started with the moms from my own loss support group, and then reached out to Anna, Margaret, and other leaders I knew in the local pregnancy-loss community. Nine other moms wanted to tell their stories. And I personally knew seven of them either from being in group with them or having spoken at one of their groups. I felt so honored that my need to share my story had also sparked others to want to tell theirs.

"Each mom e-mailed me her loss story and her SPALS story. I worked for months making suggestions for changes and editing on my own. When I knew the stories were great, I pulled other pieces together: a foreword by a prominent doctor, a synopsis chapter by a compassionate social worker, back-cover endorsements from leaders in our field, and gorgeous artwork from a friend I met on my journey.

"I began searching the Internet and the library for an agent or a publisher. Many e-mails and snail mails went unanswered, and I received several form-letter rejections as well. It was a frustrating process, and it made me wonder how any book ever got published.

"Then I thought perhaps I could get grant funding to publish it, sort of a cosponsorship with an agency. This led me to First Candle/SIDS Alliance, and while they do not offer funding, they invited me to serve on their 2005 annual conference planning committee, which I did. I was a moderator in one session, where I was able to introduce a leading doctor known to many in the prenatal loss field.

"My energy was significantly renewed after this conference, and I went home and started looking again for a way to publish my book. I came across a copublisher, someone who acts as the general manager. She read my proposal and sent me a contract of what was expected and when I had to submit it. She did a first round of editing and I was thrilled by how she streamlined the writing of the various moms. She also suggested adding a man's point of view.

"I gave first dibs to my husband, a nonwriter if there ever was one. When I read what Eric wrote, I was overwhelmed with feelings of love and forgiveness for my husband, and I knew I had made the right decision asking him to contribute. He wrote many things he could not say to me—or perhaps these were the things he always said and I just couldn't hear him. Anna can tell you: my husband is not a touchy-feely kind of guy. He handles his emotions very differently than I do, and I have often interpreted this as his not having feelings at all. But because of Eric's willingness to write about Solomon, I healed and we became closer.

"After many months and a financial investment that we knew would probably never be recouped, our book arrived in hand. Or rather, our book arrived in our driveway: thirty cartons of books that I had to haul into my house and store.

"It was exciting to see my name as editor on the cover, under the title *Journeys: Stories of Pregnancy after Loss*. We had done it. I had done it. The passionate pain and anger I had felt was now directed and molded into a book, one that would hopefully help others to heal. I immediately gave each mom who shared their story a copy of the book and sent some away for review. I set up a website and started marketing the book.

"I had been speaking at loss groups since Alison was six weeks old. It was something I felt compelled to do, and I hoped it helped others. I think it did, because I am sitting here with moms tonight whom I first met when I spoke at their loss groups. It's a very rewarding feeling for me, knowing I've helped someone enough that she, in turn, can help someone else. I don't think of myself as a leader, just as someone who is willing to share her story.

"I wanted to do a book because I felt so strongly about doing *something* in addition to speaking at the groups. I wanted to reach a larger audience, and I hope the book finds its intended readers—even though I always wish there would be no more losses. Thank you."

Anna, Margaret, and my fellow reunioners all thank me for sharing. As they speak, I can feel the differing levels of intensity among them depending on how much time has passed since their losses, and what path their healing journey had taken. Then we turn our attention to the new group members.

Mostly the women speak. But they weren't just women; they were mothers. Society may not agree with me that a woman whose baby dies before birth is now a mother, but a birth is defined as "the emergence of a new individual from the body of its parent or the act or process of bringing forth young from the womb." Why would we not refer to ourselves as mothers?

I am touched in particular by two stories. Tracy's son was born early and with undeveloped kidneys. He lived, supported in the Neonatal Intensive Care Unit (NICU), for only a few days. What brings me to tears is Tracy's description of her and her husband's families, at their sides, helping and crying and caring and nurturing Tracy. I had often felt so alone. It seemed as though the efforts anyone put out toward me were to help themselves feel better, not actually to help me. I am sure this is why I became so involved in my own support group and why I find myself repeatedly telling my story: to help others who need a connection.

Erica shares next, a story similar to my own. She lost her son during her honeymoon on a cruise ship. What strikes me is how young and collected she is, not to mention how pretty. Her husband is silently holding his wife's hand, as so many of the husbands do, as Eric did.

Even though years have passed since Solomon died, I am still surprised by how and when the grief finds me. I confide to Anna at the group's adjournment that Alex, my stepson, brought over some hand-me-down clothing for Adam, boasting, "for when he is bigger." Pulling a tie-dyed T-shirt from the bag, the breath rushed out of me and I felt my eyes start to well up with tears. It was the shirt Eric and I bought for Alex when we were on our "escape vacation," the booby-prize trip we took over the weekend of Solomon's actual due date to Washington, D.C. I carefully folded the shirt and placed it on top of the bag to show Eric. And when he came home and saw it, his only remark was "Neat shirt, cool tie-dye."

I looked at Anna and just sighed. She knows my point—she just gets it. This is the reason I continue to attend the reunion groups: to connect with those who get it. To be among peers who share a loss, to reaffirm to us that our children exist, even if they are only in our hearts.

CHAPTER NINETEEN

Standing in the Shadows of Grief

Janel C. Atlas

When I had entered the hospital just two days before, I had carried my second daughter inside my body. Now, leaving secretively through a door marked only by a small exit sign and flanked by huge trash bins, I felt drained. Around the corner stood the maternity ward main exit, where beaming new fathers held flowers while nervously adjusting the newborn car seats.

Aware of how very far I was from that door, I walked, empty-handed, to the car.

I strapped my seatbelt over my stretched-out stomach, and my husband drove us home. On the short drive, the February rush-hour traffic boggled my mind. I could not accept that people around me—people I bump into in public, people within sight of me, of the hospital where my dead daughter was born—could continue as though nothing were different. *How could they go on like nothing has changed?*

That feeling of isolation became my erstwhile companion. From the moment I learned that Beatrice had died inside of me, tangled by the umbilical cord and cut off from my body by a tightening knot, I chose loneliness.

I had assured my husband, James, that my 36-week checkup was just a routine appointment. After all, it was our second baby. He'd seen it all before—the weighing, the undressing, the measuring of the fundus. The cheerful doctor, asking how we're holding up. The predictions—so confident of the certain outcome—about when the baby would arrive.

That predictability dissolved when my doctor globbed the Doppler jelly on my belly and probed for the baby's heartbeat. Silence. He shifted position. Silence. With a look of concern on his face that quickly hardened into professional resolve, the doctor prodded the baby and tried a different angle. Silence.

I felt bile rising in my throat and waves of nausea slamming my gut. Hot tears pricked my eyes and I started to shake, the quivering of someone going into shock. He searched for what felt like an eternity but must have only been a few minutes.

I gathered my things, got dressed, and somehow managed to buckle my toddler daughter, Evelyn, into the van. The hospital was a twenty-minute drive from my obstetrician's office. Between traffic lights on a busy six-lane highway, I kept myself calm enough. But when I braked at red lights, I fell apart, crying uncontrollably. Evelyn, uncertain about what was happening, started to babble and laugh nervously. When I think back now, I wonder what other drivers thought, seeing my tears and body-racking sobs. I called my father, who was working less than an hour away, and he promised to get to the hospital as soon as he could. He told me that everything would be fine. (Dad later told me that he had been trying to calm me down so that I could drive safely. He knew what a silent Doppler meant.)

A friend met me at the hospital to care for Evelyn, and I sat to fill out maternity triage forms. By this time, I felt frozen, barely able to force my hand to check the proper boxes. "Any trouble with this pregnancy? Bleeding? Cramping? Preeclampsia?" No, no, no, no.

My husband, whom I had called before leaving the obstetrician's office, wasn't there yet, but I was so stunned that I could not delay officially receiving the news.

The maternity ward doctor put the wand to my belly, and I could immediately see what I had already known; my baby was motionless, her heart still. There were no movements, no flutters. Her heart's four tiny chambers sat open like a wound. I could see her facial profile—she looked like she was asleep.

When James hesitantly entered the examination room just a few moments later, I gathered myself enough to tell him that our baby was dead. His face split open, cracked in pain.

I watched him as they showed him our baby on the ultrasound. He saw the hopeless image of our much-desired baby, and then we clung to each other in disbelief, numb from the shock of seeing her dead but not wanting to believe it.

The medical professionals who were in the room all got teary-eyed, and one quickly walked out into the hallway, where we could hear her sobbing. We later learned that we were the third couple that week to come in to confirm a late-term fetal demise.

James and I decided to induce labor immediately, rather than go home to wait for labor to start naturally. I was wheeled up on the elevator to the maternity ward. Our first day was blessedly quiet, with only a few laboring mothers. Even so, we couldn't forget why other people were there, in that same hospital department, on the same floor. Late that night, I was awakened by the grunting shrieks of a woman in labor. The steady voice of a doctor urged her to push, and what sounded like a chorus of supporters rooted the banshee mother on. As I lay there in the dark, my hand involuntarily went to my large belly, caressing the sore ligaments along the sides. After an eternity, an eruption of cheers went up as the mother across the hall gave one last push, and I heard the squall of a brand-new baby.

I hated having to hear it. I hated that someone else's baby was fine when mine was dead. I rolled to my side, muffling my sobs with the pillow.

Waiting for the medicines to do their agonizingly slow work, my mind focused on how absurd this whole situation was. I kept saying, to myself, to visitors, to family, "This is just a sad shadow of what waiting for a baby should be." I knew the joyful sounds and bustle of a healthy birth. My first daughter had been born naturally at full term less than two years before. With that experience to look back on, I simply had never considered stillbirth.

Like so many women lucky enough to live in a country with excellent prenatal care, I had not questioned that I would bring home a healthy baby. Oh, I knew that miscarriages occurred. It was undeniably sad, but it ended in a procedure, not labor and delivery. But a baby so close to birth? Just a few weeks from the nursery, with a young, healthy mother and a beautiful older sister? It was something I had never tried to fathom.

There had been no clear signs of Beatrice's impending intrauterine death. Just the week before, at my 35-week checkup, the nurse-midwife who saw me said that I was having "a textbook pregnancy" and predicted that I would hold my baby in my arms very soon. In the moment my doctor couldn't find the heartbeat, I fell into a shadow world. As my husband and I sat awaiting Beatrice's birth, I told myself that this was a rare occurrence.

On February 9, 2006, Beatrice slid from my body with just two pushes, and the gray dawn greeted her silence with its silence. Her cord was long and silvery, shapeless. A healthy cord looks like rope, with strong bands to prevent it from looping back on itself and getting tangled. Beatrice's cord was too long, too thin, and knotted.

We left the hospital that evening, right at dusk. I couldn't bear another night listening to other babies' arrivals. I wanted to be home, and I wanted to hold my toddler tight.

Every day for the first few weeks after Beatrice's death and birth, we received cards from people all over, sending their condolences. I went out to the mailbox with a confusing mix of anticipation and dread.

Most of the cards assured us that many, many wonderful people were grieving with us and remembering Beatrice's short life. It comforted me to read the condolences. The cards and flowers covered the flat surfaces in our family room, then the dining room and kitchen. I had never received so many flowers before. *What a shame*, I remember thinking, *that my baby had to die to have a house so filled with flowers*.

Mixed in with gratitude, I felt apprehension getting the mail or answering the door because some people sent stories of friends of friends or distant family members who had experienced losses similar to mine. All of a sudden, everyone I met had a story about their sister's sister-in-law or their great-aunt or a neighbor's friend. To some mothers reeling from their babies' deaths, this might provide comfort. These stories assure newly bereaved parents that there are others who understood, who have been through it, too. Who have survived it.

To me, it didn't help to hear that I wasn't alone in my pain. I didn't want company in the shadow of my loss; I wanted to be alone in it.

Even before Beatrice's death, I wanted to be special. Even though I knew, intellectually, that there were more than four million babies born annually in the United States, I wanted to be the only one growing a baby. I was stymied by how something so everyday and so utterly mammalian could feel mystical when it happened to me. How could something so often replicated still be miraculous? When I was pregnant, I felt jealousy vibrate through me when I saw another pregnant woman.

My grief after Beatrice's death inverted this perspective. Instead of wanting to claim a monopoly on the glow of pregnancy, I wanted others to see the depth and darkness of my loss. I needed people to see how horrific, how awful it was for me to lose the baby I wanted so much so close to her due date.

So I closed my eyes and ears to stories about other people's losses. Or, when I listened, like at the support group I attended only once, my ears were attuned to the details that would help create a hierarchy of loss. Only I set out to the task already knowing that my loss was the worst.

A woman had a baby stillborn at 21 weeks. Well, that's sad, really awful. I felt for her. But her baby wasn't viable yet. My Beatrice was 36 weeks old. She was four pounds, eight ounces. She was ready to live on her own. Just the week before she died, she had a strong heartbeat.

One woman lost one twin around 20 weeks and the other survived and was born healthy at 32 weeks. I mean, that's terrible in its own way, but at least she got to bring one baby home. She's not rocking with empty arms, like I am. Her milk is feeding a baby, not streaming down her belly and down the shower drain, like mine.

I cringe admitting this ugliness. There's nothing pretty about grief, and these obsessive thoughts were compounded by the guilt I felt for thinking them. I tried to stop myself, to have grace and understanding that other people's losses did not in any way diminish mine. But it didn't work. For at least the first six months after Beatrice was born, maybe longer, I lived in a shadow. I wanted to be alone in my pain.

Looking back, I think it was necessary for me to delve into the phenomenally painful depths of Beatrice's death and the pain it caused me, even to such a degree that I mentally minimalized others' losses. Had I, in the midst of suffering such personal grief, sat with the awareness of others' equally wrenching pain, the sorrow might have overwhelmed me. So I shut it out, holding my grief close, nursing it with my tears and swaddling it in isolation.

Several years after Beatrice was stillborn, one of my dearest friends told me that she thought our similar pregnancy losses—one of her babies was found to have died at about 17 weeks and was born soon after—would connect us and draw us even closer. But at the time of Beatrice's death and for many months afterward, I drew back from her and (sometimes pointedly) communicated to her that our losses differed. I quoted the medical delineation between a miscarriage (before 20 weeks' gestation) and a stillbirth (a death anytime between 20 weeks and delivery). Even when I was saying this, my brain knew that this was an arbitrary marker—couldn't a loss at 18 weeks' gestation just as easily be called a stillbirth? Or why hadn't 23 weeks been chosen, at viability? But my grief-stained heart needed to point out the demarcation between her loss and mine.

In those first six months, instead of drawing closer to other mothers who had lost babies, I crumbled in my grief, mostly alone. Stillbirth, I told myself—and others—is a unique loss, one that cannot be understood by those outside of its shadow. Only recently did my friend and I talk about the early days after Beatrice's death, and it brought back the intense emotions of that time. I felt relief in seeing how my perspective on this has changed.

In the four years since Beatrice's death and birth, I have come to see her death as one tiny piece of the human story. It is a huge part of my story: as a person, a mother, a wife, a friend, a daughter, a writer. But the details about my pregnancy with her, the particulars about how and why she died, and the specific ways in which I grieved her have gradually faded. They've grown vague and fuzzy around the edges (I never would have believed that could happen, but it has). That's not to say that they aren't important to me and to others who loved Beatrice, who miss her now and always. But I don't cling to the specifics of the story now.

I have come through the comparing and isolation, the competitive grief I needed to live in the wake of her death. I've embraced the fact that, while the details of each loss are different, the outcome is the same: we have babies who aren't with us. My desire to define my loss as completely unique has been sated, and in its place yawns the need to be supported, surrounded, and understood by a community of families who have endured the loss of a child, whatever the details surrounding that baby's death.

Around the time of what would have been Beatrice's second birthday, I dropped off two quilts I had made at the hospital. One, about the size of a hand towel, will go to a family with a stillborn baby. The other quilt, only the size of a hot pan holder, is for a family whose baby died before 20 weeks' gestation. Both families will hold empty blankets.

I don't want these parents to leave the hospital totally empty-handed. Looking back on that frigid February evening when I left the hospital after Beatrice's birth, I know now that I was right when I thought the world was going on as it always had. It's just that I had stepped into a shadow that had always been there, just out of my view. It was only through acknowledging the presence of others there with me that I was able to step out of the darkness.

CHAPTER TWENTY

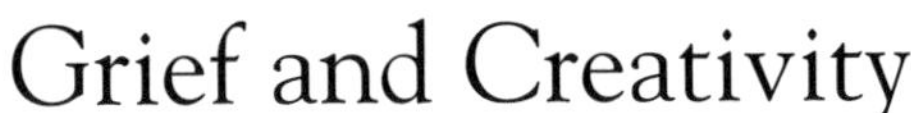

Grief and Creativity

Kara L. C. Jones

"Your baby has no heartbeat."

In the moment of trauma, everything I'd previously known was shattered into an unrecognizable mess. She said it again. "This baby has no heartbeat." And my own heart seemed to slip from its rib-cage casement and shatter across the linoleum floor. I had no idea how much creativity it would take to move from the moment of trauma, across time and space, into learning how to live life again in the face of grief and loss.

Finding the Words

> When a child dies, it is so out of the natural order that many find language fails us. In my own story and in working with other bereaved families over the years, I have seen how we are rendered speechless. Yet for all the failings of language, many of us keep reaching for a way to express the unbelievable. Some turn to art making and art sharing through programs like Laura Seftel's The Secret Club Project.[1] Others have opted to remake the language itself, as we at KotaPress have done with *The Dictionary of Loss*.[2] In whatever ways we can, bereaved parents try to understand the chaos.

As I lay in the hospital bed, a friend approached. She leaned over and placed a beautiful blank journal and a shiny, purple dream pen on the bedside table. "To put words to the chaos," she said. As thoughts dripped from my fingertips, I realized a shift had come. I was no longer writing about the childhood

I had experienced; I was writing about the childhood my son would never have. I had started to create and destroy my own myths of being; I was creatively looking at the abyss between *wanted* and *is*.

In those few hospital days and the cremation and funeral days following, I began to notice time was functioning differently than it had before. While time seemed to flow in a linear fashion for those around us, time in our household meandered through a mixed-up maze of past, present, and future. The dark hallway leading from the bedroom to the living room seemed like a portal to a foreign land where I no longer had a name. I was not a mother, as I had no physical child to signify my parenthood. I was denied a birth certificate, as if the slice from hip to hip did not count as giving birth. I was, however, given a death certificate, as if to confirm I was indeed a freak who had given birth to death, not my son. It became very real, very fast. I realized I would forever be looking askew at my own life. We would never again walk within the halls of society's generalized definition of "normal."

Friends who could not face their own mortality issues vanished. My husband's then-employer became a heartless dictator who rang our home and actually said, "Well, it isn't like you brought a baby home, so we don't understand why you can't come back to work." And older women—complete strangers—approached us in public after we shared our story, saying things like "My own son died the same way fifty years ago, and I've never been allowed to say his name out loud."

Amid the chaos, there was only one safe and sacred space I could go to express what was happening for me in any given moment: creativity. Not only the creativity of writing and drawing, but the creativity it took to figure out why I should get out of bed every morning when I woke with a rush of memory and the pull of an abdomen wound telling me, yes, indeed, it was real. He was dead. I was a childless mother.

Breaking the Silence

> In doing grief and creativity work, a recurring theme I see is families living in fear that their children will be forgotten, the dead child's name lost to silence. Some combat this by writing their child's name in the sand or wearing a bracelet made of lettered beads to spell out the name. These are creative acts of nonviolent protest, expressions of committed love. These parents are telling the world, "Silence will not be tolerated."

Prior to his death, I considered myself an academic poet. I knew what it meant to write, attend workshops, endure critiques to the point of having a wholly different poem, rework it, and spend countless stamps ponying the work around, hoping some editor would publish it without asking for yet more changes. But the pieces I was writing after his death were all I had left of my baby. How in the world could I take him into critique circle and let them kill him again? How in the world could I send him off to some strange editor who would think he knew best how to present my baby to the reader? I began to dread the process, but I also felt fearful that I would never be published again because I would not abide the rules of the academic game any longer. I didn't fit anywhere anymore. My previous life was truly destroyed in every way.

As I lamented this to my partner, Hawk, he prodded me, "Why don't we just publish it ourselves?" and "Why do you have to send it off to anyone?" The academic in me screamed that to skirt the respected avenues to publication would equate to vanity. But the heARTist in me felt her asthma attack recede as air rushed in, allowing her to dream again. I got even more excited when Hawk suggested we name our press Kota, in honor of our son's name, Dakota. I imagined answering the phone in the future, saying my son's name out loud: "KotaPress. How may I help you?" His name would not be lost to the silence of a tombstone or a dusty, aging, unfinished baby book after all. And I was completely sold when we came up with the acronym KOTA: Knowing Ourselves Thru Art. So of course, we should just publish my poems ourselves. I was becoming a different kind of poet and a Different Kind of Parent.[3]

A Tangible Parenthood

The invisibility of being a childless parent poses a lifelong challenge for the bereaved. If we have other children, visibility of the full scope of our parenthood is still an issue. Surviving siblings miss brothers and sisters who are never seen by teachers and friends. Grandparents know with every visit that a loved family member is missing. Because our experiences lack tangibility, creativity—the gift of using our hands—can bless our lives. As Cathy A. Malchiodi wrote in the *Art Therapy Sourcebook*, "Art therapy is perhaps one of the few therapies in which you create a tangible product." As such, via creativity, families like ours can make parenthood tangible. It might be as simple as an ornament on the Christmas tree featuring the name of the child who died. Or a random act of kindness done anonymously, but a Kindness Card[4] left to say that the action was done in the name of the child. Or making sure Mother's and Father's days include all the parents present at your celebration; if flowers are being given to parents of living children, we make sure childless parents also receive flowers.

Not only did I not have a physical baby to signify my parenthood, but also the continual minimization of our experience drove me with fire and passion in those early days of grief. I became determined to break the cycle of invisibility. I remembered vividly the prenatal appointments when health care providers asked for my family history to assess possible risks to me, the pregnancy, Dakota. I thought I didn't have any to share. But then, days after Kota's death, suddenly I found myself a part of conversations that ended with things like, "Your sister's first baby was stillborn," or "Your aunt lost several babies before her daughter was born," or "Your Nona had more than one child who died as a baby." The silence surrounding those children's deaths had robbed me of my full medical and family history. Would the knowledge of these things have changed anything in my pregnancy with Dakota? No one can say. But at the very least, we all deserve to know our medical histories. On that idea alone, I refused to be silent.

The other force that drove me to creative, tangible expression was how the silence and invisibility worked so quickly to cut us off from the world at large. How could I reconnect with the people in my neighborhood, even? One day I was pregnant and excited. The next day, my round baby bump was obviously gone, so people asked, "Where is that precious baby?" When I answered with tears—or worse yet, raging anger—or uttered the words, "Our baby died," you can imagine the stunned silences.

The conversations we had with our caregivers were also part of what set me on my radically creative path. Almost immediately upon Dakota's death, we heard things like, "This so rarely happens," and "You can try again," and "Statistically this almost never happens twice." While I understood that the speakers had good hearts and good intentions, I felt the experience we were having with our current child, with this present birth and death, was being minimized.

With all that in mind, we started KotaPress, and launched into having our first two books, *Flash of Life* and *Mrs. Duck and the Woman*, put into print. To me, the creative act of bringing the books to print was my first product of visible, tangible parenthood. We had sponsors for those first print runs, so we were able to give away several hundred copies of the books directly to bereaved families, caregivers, hospitals, doctors' offices, and midwives' birthing centers. When we approached our own caregivers about how many books they might want in their office, they told us ten copies would be a lot because, again, "this so rarely happens." And they added, "In fact, in twenty years of practice, your family was our first stillbirth." I took a deep breath, smiled, thanked them, and left ten copies. Six months later, the phone rang; it was one of the doctors from the same office. She opened her call with an apology to me. She was calling to request more copies of the books. Stunningly, in that six-month period, they had seen so many losses that all ten books were given away to bereaved families already. My heart broke for those families, and at the same time, I felt great appreciation for the sponsors who made those books available for families to have validation of their experiences.

This was becoming our way of reconnecting to the world at large. As families around the globe received copies of our books, we got e-mails and phone calls of thanks, requests for additional copies, and interest in finding out more about our work at KotaPress. Hawk and I were just starting to figure out that this was going to be our life's work. The love, time, money, and energy we would have devoted to Kota would now go to this work. We were finding a new tribe, a new place in the world, a new way to define ourselves.

Patience in the Impatient World

> Rollo May wrote in the book *The Courage to Create*, "The creative process must be explored not as a product of sickness but as representing the highest degree of emotional health, as the expression of normal people in the act of actualizing themselves." The actualization of bereaved parents is unique from person to person, as each of us comes to terms with what happened. It takes a great deal of time and patience—while living in this impatient world—to remake the meaning of being alive, risking to love in the face of death, fully discovering who we are now that grief has ravaged all previous definitions of self. For some, this redefinition will include things like remaking the holidays as less about gift-giving and more about volunteering or making donations to people and organizations in need. For others, the actualization can be as comprehensive as giving up previous work to start a new career. Whatever the creative changes we undergo, they are part of a lifelong process. The bereaved must learn to be gentle with themselves throughout all of this—because often the impatient world stands, tapping its foot, waiting for them to "get over it."

As the people in our everyday lives got impatient with how we were sinking our money and time into this new business that, in their eyes, kept us stuck in grief, we were just beginning to understand how our lives had changed. Many of our friends and loved ones seemed to hold onto an expectation of a time when we would "get back to normal." While I could never get anyone to explicitly tell me what that meant, my intuition told me people were impatient for us to return to some kind of pre-death version of ourselves. It was difficult to explain to people that a return was simply never going to happen. Our everyday consciousness now includes Dakota's death, and mortality in general. Dakota's death shook to the core whatever faith we previously had. Our son stays with us, even in my physical body. At least, I sensed that.

Confirmation came when I read about research in the *Journal of the American Medical Association*. The researchers discovered that fully functioning cells of every baby stay in the mother's body.[5] The baby's cells last long, long after the pregnancy ends, regardless of whether the pregnancy ends in a live birth or a stillbirth. This research paper confirmed for me that I am, even down to the cellular level, changed by my son's presence in my life, in my body.

In this breakdown of all we had previously known, in the dismantling of every boundary we had ever placed on ourselves, we were making the most creative choices we could. We were attending to ourselves. While reading the *Art Therapy Sourcebook*, I learned that the Greek word *therapia* means "to be attentive to." I experienced an epiphany: that is what we were doing—a self-therapy of sorts. Once the shock of death wore off, we came back into our disjointed selves and chose to practice creativity as a way to re-create our lives. Again in the *Art Therapy Sourcebook*, Cathy A. Malchiodi writes that for those "who have experienced the death of a significant person, the act of making art is a way of remaking the self after loss." This is exactly what we were doing with KotaPress.

Connecting with other bereaved families through our work with KotaPress enabled us to reconnect with the world at large, yet within the context of our new identities. Unlike the people in our everyday lives who could not make sense of what we were doing, the readers of our books accepted us exactly as we defined ourselves now. As we increased our community connections by working with organizations like the MISS Foundation, we found spaces where we could be ourselves entirely. Attending our first MISS conference, I was struck by how easy it was to laugh. I could laugh without anyone jumping to the conclusion that I had finally recovered or was "better now." I could cry in the very next moment without anyone heaving a heavy sigh as if to scold, "Geesh, I thought you were better." Being in community with other bereaved families meant spending time with people who understood how very long the reintegrative process takes. Every single one of them understood that not only would the winter holidays be different this year, but also that they would be different every year for the rest of our lives.

With these affirmations buoying me along, I started learning to be patient with myself in this impatient world. I began to verbalize what I needed in my everyday life. Friends were hesitant to invite me to baby showers for friends, but if they excluded me, I got upset. So I finally began just saying, "I want to be invited so I feel included," but in the next breath, "I want you to understand I will probably decline the invitation." This was the paradox of my reality now. If friends wanted to stay in communication with me, then this grief duality was part of the deal.

I practiced patience by doing everyday things, like going to work and doing errands. Yes, the errands still had to be done. If I found myself at the post office and suddenly there was a family so precious that all the customers started cooing over the little ones, I allowed myself to simply walk away and go home. Yes, working was necessary so that we could do basic things like make ends meet. But I envisioned what it would be like to go back to an office. I'd be stuck in a place where everyone around me had photos of their babies on their desks and cubicle walls. I imagined putting a photo of my son on my desk, too. I envisioned being pulled aside by a boss or HR person and being informed that other employees didn't like seeing death up close and personal. I pictured responding that I didn't like seeing their lives either. The whole thing would come down to office policy. If family pictures were allowed, then all family pictures were allowed, period. Otherwise, it is discrimination. Talk about a bumpy reintegration vision!

So I had to learn to be patient with myself in redefining how we earn our livelihood. Back before it was fashionable, we chose telecommuting work and freelance work. We found ways to do commercial art via the press as well as our expressive arts outreach. Even now, more than a decade later, it doesn't provide six-figure incomes or reliable health care, but it keeps us reconnecting with the world at large and living our everyday lives in as radically creative a way as possible.

A Radical Creativity

> As Eugene J. Mahon wrote in his essay "The Death of Hamnet: An Essay on Grief and Creativity," "The complexity of creativity can never be reduced to a single genetic source . . . [but] the deepest sorrow can be transformed into beauty when indomitable genius insists on transcending its own suffering." I see this insistent, indomitable genius in almost every bereaved parent I meet. Whether it is finding gentle, loving, and creative ways to tell subsequently born siblings about the big brother who died, or giving up everything to go back to school to enter the caregiving professions, these parents are striving to transcend what has happened. Note that I am not talking about "getting over it" or "having closure." Rather, it's about integrating the experiences of death and grief in order to make radically creative lives for themselves.

Creativity became a practice for me, an insistence, really. Just as others might practice yoga at sunrise every day, little by little, making one small creative choice after another, suddenly I was leading an entirely creative life. A creative life, born from the urgent fire of grief.

At first I wondered if this was an oddity, if maybe I was denying the reality of what had happened to our family. To my wonder, I began to meet person after person, all bereaved parents, working with exactly this same kind of insistent energy. Dr. Joanne Cacciatore, who founded MISS after her daughter Cheyenne died. Laura Seftel, who founded The Secret Club Project after her own miscarriage and learning of her family history, which included deaths she'd never heard about prior to her own loss. Filmmaker Vanessa Gorman, who shared her daughter's birth and death with us in the stunning film *Losing Layla*. Liz Allen, who, after the death of her daughter Janell, founded the Small Victory Project, which provided CARE kits to parents and hospitals for many years. Lorraine Ash, who wrote the book *Life Touches Life* after the death of her daughter Victoria and learning of a family history of stillbirth and miscarriage. Paula Long, who founded Honored Babies after the death of her son Kadin. Cheryl Haggard, who founded Now I Lay Me Down to Sleep after the death of her son Maddux. There are dozens, hundreds, thousands more stories like these. I meet new families every single day, and their stories continue to confirm that this insistent creativity is not odd at all. Rather, we are all remaking our communities, one creative step at a time. We are remaking ourselves.

For me personally, the first acts of re-creation were all about the words that came when we first started KotaPress. On the website, I wrote and shared articles every time some new grief issue came to my awareness. In print, I shared ideas for finding our way, comparing our pre-death and post-death lives, helping others put their words into print. But there were also times when the linear nature of language just could not touch my story. So my creative insistence began looking for other means of expression.

In 2002, when words failed me, I decided to take a bookmaking class. While I found it interesting to learn about the exactness of binding, I was also intrigued to learn of more artful, guerrilla, handmade books like those of Ed Hutchins. Ed inspired me to begin thinking more sculpturally about bookmaking, and one day I happened upon the idea of a womb book. I took one of those wavy paper crates that grocery stores used to hold apples, and I cut it up so there were two waves for each book. I folded that in half, which gave me a shape representing Womb. Then I stitched the fold together using coarse string and painted the whole thing with a thick red acrylic paint, inside and out. Using a red silk string I made a long umbilical cord that tied deep within the wave covers and came out to attach to a small accordion-fold book in the shape of DaVinci's "Study of a Womb" image. The cord was very long, so that it could wrap around the book to keep it closed. But it also represented my own son's cord death. I used a delicate rice paper for the guts of the book and hand-stamped, "Without my consent / Birthing death / Womb grave" along with abbreviations for statistics like height, weight, length, name. I made seven copies of the Womb Book to display at an art gallery. The opening night event was scheduled to last two hours. Statistically speaking, 3.5 babies are stillborn every hour of every day in the United States. So the seven books represented the seven babies who would die while we all looked at art for two hours on opening night.

After that event, I made other books, but there were times again when the structure of bookmaking failed me as a means of expression. And so I turned to things like intuitive painting, scribbling to self-assess, and Artist Trading Cards (ATCs). ATCs were one of the most intriguing ideas, because their creation allowed me to trade my art with others. As I got familiar with how art swaps work, I ventured into hosting my own swaps. I looked for small groups of other bereaved parents who might want to explore making art and trading to share our stories. In 2009 we hosted a Day of the Dead heART Swap that included parents from all over the world, making art unique to their family's experience of child death. We were so moved by the exchange that we did a full, professional photo shoot to create a free e-book to share. As readers have discovered it, they've responded by asking how they too can participate in future swaps. The insistence beats on throughout the bereaved community.

Again, in my own personal process, when the insistence of swaps failed to fully touch what I was experiencing, I explored other tools like henna body art, Reiki, and Tapping/Emotional Freedom Technique for integration of experiences. All of these tools have become part of an everyday practice for me.

It's Called a Practice, Not a Perfect.

Cathy A. Malchiodi wrote in the *Art Therapy Sourcebook*, "Art therapy is a dynamic therapy, requiring one to participate in one's own treatment, in this case through making art. Therefore, truly understanding art therapy requires firsthand experience." And the same can be said for learning to live a radically creative life in the face of death, grief, and loss. In my own life and in working with others, I discovered that radical creativity is a choice to participate in our own stories, to reengage, to keep having firsthand experiences with alternative options for expressing grief, over long periods of time. For some, this flies in the face of what their everyday community is telling them. Many feel pressured to find a kind of closure that is imposed upon bereaved parents. Family and friends, sometimes even caregivers, make indications that there is some-

> thing wrong with us if we are still exploring grief a decade after our child has died. In working with families, I try to help people see that just as the parent of a living child will be a parent forever, with evolving roles and changing expressions of that parenthood as their child grows, so too, will the bereaved parent forever explore his or her role. Our relationship and expression of grief and our different kind of parenthood will change and evolve for the rest of our lives.

A few years after our son died, I was lamenting to a yogi friend, Mekosun, that I was not getting over this grief in the ways everyone around me seemed to want. He smiled at me and said my path was much like the yoga path. It's about honoring a practice, not a perfect. I felt a rush of relief at hearing his words. This was not about finding a way to be perfectly healed, to lead a pre-death life again, nor about living in ways others predefined for me. Rather, this was a practice of creativity. This was a continual choice to feel what I feel when I feel it, allowing for experimentation with and expression of my truth in any given moment, so I could integrate this always-evolving, radical new reality.

As I did this in my own life, people began asking me to help them learn to tap into their creativity, too. I began what amounts to a person-centered approach, in the practice of working with others. In my work with other bereaved people, I offer lots of ideas, options, tools to try. People are trying on possibilities, and I let them explore for themselves, supporting them as they find a right fit for their individual lives. It is amazing how the simple act of hosting a permissive space for another can help shift his or her entire view of grief and post-death life experiences.

Always in this work, I keep in my heART what Dr. Peter Barr told me when I first met him at a MISS Foundation conference: "There is no prescription for grief." I have learned, and continue to teach others, that there is simply no right or wrong way to experience this kind of grief; no single answer fits every person. It seems to me that all of us—bereaved parents, family, friends, and professional caregivers—would do well, would serve each other in much healthier ways, if we could all just remember this. Be gentle with each other instead of demanding. Foster patience in the impatient world. I, for one, know that as a fellow bereaved parent and as a caregiver, I must honor this pledge. I have been given a gift, and for the rest of my life, I will continue to help people find their own unique, creative ways to move from the moment of trauma, across space and time, into learning how to live life again in the face of mortality, loss, and grief.

CHAPTER TWENTY-ONE

The Year of Angels

Suzanne Pullen

Poetry allows us to bypass our brains and reach into the most visceral feelings of the moment. I have written many times about my loss, as a journalist for a magazine, as an academic for research, and as a playwright for the stage. But always, always, the first time my pen touches paper, it is as poetry. Poetry is the way I first see my inner self moving outside my body. It is the way I begin to know, to unpack, to make real, what no one else can see. Poems are written in the moment, to capture the moment. They are immediate and unapologetic in form. They are the seeds for everything I have written since . . . they are the touchstones I return to . . . to remind me that what I felt was real.

These poems, along with a few journal entries and e-mails, were my guardian angels guiding me through the darkest and most beautiful year of my life.[1]

First Trimester (The Start of Something Big . . .)

December 13, 2004
Something New

Words   coming slow
Waiting to be born
Nine months of thought
before nib touches paper

Waiting for time to resume a course meant for me

Waiting for growing anticipation
to yield past
the doubt and worry
of what won't be
rather than being open and yielding to what is

Searching for words
to touch deep
to penetrate

Stopping short by the words
that filled the pages of so many other poems

Stopped short by unfamiliar territory
not knowing how to grasp
this new metaphor
I have no vocabulary
for the baby that grows
inside a bubble devoid of language

I have no control over this process
waiting   time   ticking
my body bringing life
As hundreds of thousands die
by war and disease
anger and hate

This small miracle
        working behind the scenes
Beneath my belly
        (under cover)
Growing   stretching   moving
A small gift of magic
In an untamable sea

I am not the one saying Yes!   or   NO

This creation grows inside
needing no words
to guide synapses
or spark wonder

or describe sensations
or taste beauty
or shape the color of need

The seed growing inside my belly
has a vocabulary of its own

Spelling out fingers
and skin
and eyes
and limbs
and organs
knitting together life

My body will create
the greatest poem I have ever written
without any of the words
I have learned to say were mine

Second Trimester (Doing It Together)

December 20, 2004
To: Trish
From: Suzanne

Hey Mamacita! I made it past the first trimester! Had another ultrasound and everything looks good. Due Date: June 19, 2005, Father's Day. Just six more months to go . . . I think it is so amazing that we are doing this at the same time! Two very different ways of conceiving . . . two very different intentions . . . two different kinds of parental units . . . but two amazing women doing something more amazing than we may realize.

To: Suzanne
From: Trish

Hola Chicita—

I'm so glad to hear that everything is OK and that Boo Boo is well. I am still convinced something is wrong or that I've miscarried. I am so anxious for my ultrasound on the 15th. I doubt I'd be this worried if I hadn't have gone through lots of $$ and time and anguish for 2+ years, but there's so much at stake that I'm stressed!

You'll have to update me on everything when you visit. We can talk "baby talk" for hours and we won't bore our friends who think we're nuts.

February 14, 2005
Beyond Worry

For the last 5½ months
My left hand on my belly
My brain on worry and future plans
No word from the baby daddy
After being clear that I wanted nothing from him
Out of shame
Or guilt
Or obligation

Now I am moving through
The uncertainty of these words
Not ashamed at being 35
Single
And pregnant
But full of shame in his being the father
My son will be the third generation without one

Constant battles between doubt and knowingness
At war with enjoying this moment
Diving into a deep blue tar pit
Of regurgitated resentment
Traced with whispers of wonder
And sinking deeper into the truth
I know is at the center
A diamond made by my spirit
My soul
My magic
Beyond my worry

February 19, 2005
Stages of Joy

Moving furniture
Shifting organs
Clearing out worries
Settling into peace
Needing all nine months
to prepare for this life altering life giving

There are the five stages of grief
As there are the five stages of this joy
Physical anxiety
    —will my body reject this seed

Mental anxiety
—will I make enough money to help the seed grow
Preparation
—make lists and check them twice
Stages four and five
Are what the future holds
I'll tell you how to get to nirvana
When this baby is born.

Unexpected Outcomes

March 01, 2005
9:30 a.m.
His heart stopped beating

10:45 p.m.
You don't get the baby's cry at the end of this road
Another gift awaits you
Let go
Let go
Open open open

You have an amazing body
You can do this
Avery's already on the Good Road . . .

. . . you need to send his body home . . .

March 03, 2005
2:34 a.m.
Avery (leader of the elves) Pullen was born

9:30 a.m.
I said good-bye as they took his body away

11:30 a.m.
Not sure I am ready to write it yet
But not wanting to forget
Needing to remember every moment with him
after opening the door in my body
the house he lived in
Opening to the Good Road

Willing my body to let go
before it was ready
willing him to leave this casket
from a womb
Against every instinct my body knew

Friends just barely planning his house warming
now standing as midwives
to him moving out
My hands holding my belly
sending love and energy for 6 months
Now spurring contractions with each touch
laboring without the promise of the present
at the end

Every child's birthright
but mine
a gift
given too soon

Just like that
It was over
After 31 hours of labor
Less than 10 hours from the news
9:30 a.m. Tuesday to 2:30 a.m. Thursday

And yet when he came
a small treasure
cradled between my breasts
and tucked under my chin

I can still feel the weight of him
so much more than the pound and a half in my hand

5:30 p.m.

Things to remember:

> Feeling his soft cool head against my chest
> His long perfect hand draped across my finger
> His big feet
> Toes like mine and his grandmom's
> Tacky skin slick with his waters
> 13 inches long

Ruby Red Lips
Smelling powdery sweet
Both of us being held by infinity   family and friends

StasSamAnnaBeckyMomJenKalaDrissanaHeatherJasonErin

The doctor I met just that day saying:

"It isn't often we get to give birth to angels here . . ."

before she left the room so I wouldn't see her cry

11:30 p.m.

My son . . .
Is still too big to fit onto pages this small
So grateful to have had this chance
So unsure of where to go from here

My life changed 6 months ago
And now my life has changed again
    So suddenly
Midwifed through the birth of death

Afterbirth

March 08, 2005

7:30 a.m.

Watching the full-grown sandpipers
Realizing my life has been all about

    . . . waiting
Making due with the   in between   time
Making things happen while waiting
for my dream to come true.
Waiting for the man in my lighthouse dream to come
Made this baby and
suddenly
this waiting had an end
8 months
then 7
then 6
The Universe gave me a due date when my waiting would be over

And now
I am back to waiting again
        Back to
Square One
Day One
with the numbers counting up instead of down

Watching the waves
scatter pipers
just feet from me
Seeing for the first time in all my years of watching
the white and black wingspan as they take flight

Understanding that beautiful things come
during the waiting

These are the things
I wanted to show him . . .
. . . the sun rising over the dunes
casting morning gold through the sea grass
. . . the pipers' fast straw feet racing away from bubbling foam
. . . the ocean's power thundering a steady pulse

I can only see so much with these eyes
desperate to share this world's beauty

Left instead waiting
wading in time
closing my eyes

So I can see him again

March 10, 2005

Voicemail from Trish:

"Suzanne, it's Trish."

She's sobbing . . . OH NO . . . please . . . NOT HER BABY TOO . . .

"I just read your e-mail."

Oh thank goodness . . .

"I'm so sorry."

Her sobs get louder . . .

"I feel so awful. I can't imagine . . ."

No . . . she can't . . . but she understands, in a way none of my other friends can, what I have lost . . .

March 21, 2005

Spring Equinox
Once growing womb-belly
full minded
working overtime
worry worry   worry

Now belly emptying
sorrow growing
losing him too soon
wanting what I couldn't have

Standing in a hot shower I'msorry I'msorry I'msorry I'msorry
I'msorry I'msorry I'msorry I'msorry I'msorry I'msorry
I'msorry I'msorry I'msorry I'msorry I'msorry I'msorry I'msorry
IamsosorryIamsosorryIamsosorryIamsosorryIamsosorryIamsosorry until the words
and tears and water feel as cold as the ache that sobs my body to sleep

    Passing between the worlds
to birth the death   of a future
no longer viable
membranes thick with grief
    A very deep wound
My womb
from a gift to a grave

March 22, 2005

To: Trish
From: Suzanne

Hey—

I'm here in Arizona . . . doing as you'd expect . . . except that my mom has so opened up since Avery died . . . she is truly undergoing an emotional transformation . . . she never got to hold her first baby who she said died in an incubator . . . it's like having held Avery is helping heal a 40-year-old wound . . .

I was so glad we spent some time together last week. Thank you for giving me permission to always share my feelings about Avery . . . It's hard, but I really want to try to be present for you and your baby, so let's keep working through this together . . .

OK . . . how am I doing?

This is the hardest thing I've ever had to go through . . . hard because it is too easy to pick up my life and put one foot in front of the other . . . because that's just what I do. I'll laugh at my mother and Jen teasing each other. Drink in the sweet smell of orange blossoms in my parents' back yard. Watch rabbits rise up on their hind legs to eat the new growth at the bottom of the trees.

And then I will remember I was supposed to be preparing to share all of this with a growing bundle of magic inside me . . . a gift that I had to give back . . . and it seems so unimaginable that my life has changed all over again and so suddenly. I want everything to stop . . . everything is different now. The tears feel like the first time every time.

And then I see a picture of him . . . and I know that he was here . . . and he was real. And my body made him. And the gifts that he gave me are worth all the sadness in me . . .

And one day, I hope, magic will happen again in my womb . . . and I will be able to tell the story of a little brother that opened a door to my heart and made room in my house for a new hope to grow.

To: Suzanne
From: Trish

Hey Suzanne—

Good to hear from you. I'm glad you've taken some time for yourself to truly grieve and to heal. So many times people just sweep their feelings under the rug and don't deal with them; then they resurface through unhealthy ways. I'm glad your mom is sharing an emotional transformation with you and that you are handling Avery's gifts and emptiness.

April 15, 2005
Rage

It isn't the autopsy report
That breaks me down

It's seeing the woman across from me
          Rub her belly

It isn't seeing the dome of the columbarium
          (Where I picked up Avery's ashes)
Framed by the doctor's window
while my feet are freezing in stirrups

It's hearing another baby's heart beating
from the Doppler next door.

It isn't that people see me cry so much
It's that no one realizes that in the silence
I am still screaming

May 08, 2005
These Hands

I have been so ANGRY at my hands
Hours spent
consciously and unconsciously sending love and Reiki
into my belly
but it wasn't enough
to keep Boo Boo's heart beating

These hands *betrayed* me
I HATE THEM!!!!!!!!!!!!!!!!!!!!!!!!
Why didn't they tell me something was wrong . . . .

I haven't touched my belly since he left

I ask the masseuse to heal my hands
but they are just the symptom
She holds them lightly
and I move between the worlds
I hear a voice in my head like an angel

"Listen to these hands. These hands spoke to him. He is still alive in these hands. Listen to these hands."

I hear on NPR (not long after) that fetal cells stay inside the mother's body
for months
sometimes years
after her pregnancy
it doesn't matter if the baby was miscarried, terminated, or full term
these cells are present at sites of disease and illness

not to make the mother sick
but to help her heal
Maybe there is still a part of him inside of me . . .
. . . still alive
. . . healing my hands

Maybe this is why we still feel our babies with us . . . because a part of them still is . . .

(date unknown days run together coming too fast to the end)

Stas and Anna tell me:

> Hasidic tradition says that from the time your child is conceived, he is not alone.
>
> A guardian angel stays in the womb with him as he grows, teaching him everything he needs to
> know about life and love. Teaches him about his purpose
> and how to be a good person.
>
> Just as the bag of waters breaks, before your child is born, the angel shouts, "WAIT!"
> She reaches out her finger, touches the space between his nose and lip and says, "So you forget."
> And he comes crying into the world, only to have to learn everything all over again.
>
> If that is true, then for the babies who
> died before they were born,
> their angel never reached out to touch the space between their nose and lip.
> They remembered everything.
> About life. About love.
> About you.

I never got to look into Avery's eyes or into his soul or learn what kind of person he was going to become. So I have a hard time imagining him looking down over me from wherever his energy may, or may not, be swirling. But with those words, I see him rushing off with all the hope and love I had for him filling his little spirit. I can imagine him feeling my heart beat for him and I can believe that he felt truly wanted. He took the only gifts I could give him and brought them with him on the Good Road.

June 09, 2005

To: Trish

From: Suzanne

I have been trying to send you an e-mail all week . . . but my fingers keep freezing at the keyboard. They also froze every time I tried to pick up the phone on Saturday to send you my best wishes during your shower. Thank you for understanding why it was just too hard to be there . . .

I love you, Trish. And I have nothing but the deepest love for you and your baby.

I look forward to getting to know him and giving you whatever support I can offer,

Suzanne

To: Suzanne
From: Trish

Heyya Girl—

Been thinking about you lots too. The shower Saturday was very nice—lots of people and great energy. Jayden Michael Tin Law is expected on July 1st, 2005, by C-section! Jayden means "ball of fire." Michael means "god-like" (after my father); Tin means "sky" in Chinese (after Jayden's grandfather—his middle name). As my dad says, we're having a "god-like ball of fire from the sky"! Look out! Tomorrow is my last day at work and I'm exhausted trying to wrap things up not only for the year, but also for the 6 months I'll be out in the fall.

Take care of yourself as the June days go by . . . I'm here for you too.

Trish

Due Dates

June 19, 2005
The Due Date

Wading through days
In another waiting pattern
    Waiting for his due date
Before I can resume a life without him.
Time is a strange companion
Weeks fly by
    Days . . . . . . drag

I can't believe it was this long before he was supposed to be born.
I don't want it to be his due date yet . . . I'm not ready for this to be over

I want a sign
I need him to help me get ready for this
Returning to the retreat center where I had been the week before he died
crying to the masseuse my need to prepare to say good-bye again
She whispers in my ear:
"Allow yourself to sink into the table and listen to the crashing of the waves.
Allow the sorrow to come and the beauty . . . because it is there, too."

Drifting in and out of bliss
    When the masseuse puts her hands on my heart and belly

The voice of my angel drifts into my head:

"I love you, Mama.
I love you for wanting me so much.
I love you for feeling so sad.
I love you for loving me.
I love you even though I couldn't stay."

Tears streaming
I am wrapped in a calm like a blanket
My mind doesn't care where the words came from,
my heart was open enough to hear them.
My feet beginning to feel the first footsteps on a new journey
I know I am on the Good Road
        Because hope isn't about waiting.
It's about the magic in the making

June 25, 2005

To: Suzanne
From: Trish

One week left . . .

What miracles you and I have been blessed with bringing into this world at a not-so-coincidental time! Our journeys, each with their own challenges and triumphs, have forever intertwined us and our two little sweethearts together in creating and experiencing family. Thank you for standing with open arms in the possibility of your son, Avery . . . for being open, giving, loving, to all that he's offered you . . . and for sharing it with me. It has taught me so much.

When I think about being a mother, I sometimes panic about how much I have to learn . . . I worry that I won't be "good enough" . . . and then I think of you and your little angel, Avery, and all that you learned from him. And I remember that it's not at all about me "doing" anything—it's about me being: being open to the joys, frustrations, and possibilities that Jayden will teach me. I hope this gift reminds you of your Baby Being . . . of your Angel Avery. Know that he has taught me much.

You are an amazing spirit . . . an amazing mother.

With love, Trish.

To: Trish
From: Suzanne

I LOVE THE ANGEL CHARM!

I put it on the bracelet Renita gave me this morning next to the charm of Avery's footprint . . . it is perfect . . . and I love that you looked for so long and wanted to find something precious for me. The timing of the giving was perfect too . . .

I take a small bit of solace in knowing that life continues to grow inside of you . . . I look forward to holding him in my arms, looking into his eyes and telling him what amazing parents he has . . . .

I can't believe you are just weeks away from completing an adventure I so wish I would have been able to see to the finish in the way I expected. I would have him in my arms now and I would be telling you all the things to expect . . .

A part of me has been holding my breath for you and the life that you have worked so hard to bring this far. The other part of me sees my little elf curled up in your belly, whispering all the things Avery learned into Jayden's ear.

July 05, 2005
To: Suzanne
From: Trish

It was so great to see you at the hospital. Thank you so much for coming and thank you for the pictures. I love that you got one of Jayden looking up at you. He didn't open his eyes for many people (still doesn't) . . . he must have known you were Avery's mom . . .

I had a dream last night that during my C-section the doctors told me I was having twins. First they pulled out Jayden.

The second baby was Avery.

Trish

The Road Ahead

December 2005
The Secret Club

We come together
across continents
and cultures
In support groups
at memorials
across kitchen tables
through hospitals
on websites

We are strangers
instantly familiar
Our number vast
and unknowable

Some meeting in person
others inducted in absentia

Broken open
Our futures ripped apart
So that our stories
pour out in blood
and tears
into a stone soup
made
when we thought
we could never be hungry
again

And once we'd wrung our bitterness dry
reduced our mingled grief over a burning ache
We looked down into a clear broth
and found the beautiful bounty
our children left us
Their gift to us so bright and brilliant
It will shine through us
until we, too, are gone

We are the proud members
of a Secret Club
We all paid a high price
for exclusive rights
To speak the names of our babies
when the condolence cards
no longer come
To weep uncontrollably
in grocery stores
when a memory steals our breath
To at once fear anniversaries and holidays
while revering the one day
meant just for them

And to risk breaking open
all over again
by loving ourselves
our families
our friends
even while we are consumed

with a desperate desire
to hold another child
in our arms again

We occasionally allow others
to observe our proceedings—
The ignorant ones, who say things like
"In time you'll get over it,"
and the dear ones who send a card
every year on the right day
and never ask why
you still cry

And we regretfully hold a place for new members
Keep a space warm and ready for their raw wounds
to be witnessed
and seen
and honored
So that there is always one place they can go
where everyone understands
without ever having to say a word
So that the world can stop for them
until they are ready to move again

Because eventually everyone in the Secret Club
folds back into a world forever changed
Even the most reticent of us
learns how to be a part
of the forward momentum required
of living things
and as loving parents we know
our love is not defined by our pain
—our love is strengthened by it.

Some of us will seem as if we can't forget
—we just aren't afraid of remembering
Others of us will seem "normal"
—it's easier for some to think of us that way
Some of us will raise a call to action
—we see what went wrong and want to make it right
Some of us will weave words into memorials
—because our babies were the most beautiful poems we ever wrote

And some of us will help the world remember
the gift our babies were in our lives
even if they never took a breath
—Because not a single one of us will ever forget

Epilogue

October 03, 2006
Something New—Part Two

Words coming slow
not knowing how to be born

An eternity of loss
before this pen
could even begin to touch this paper

Waiting for confidence
to grow past the worry and doubt
of what was the last time
instead of
what is and can be
this time

Again making life
This time an active determined choice
In spite of the unforgiving mystery
that took my first blessing
much too soon

Now creating an even bigger miracle
working under the scenes
growing
stretching
moving

Giving me the gift of trust to cling to
in an uncertain sea of panic

Some days my grip loosens
and my head dips below the surface
and my mind begins to pound with "what-if's"

And air escapes my nose in a tumble of
"Don't want this too much"

"Don't get too comfortable"
"Don't believe your wish will come true,
or when his heart stops beating
yours will break all over again."

And just as the spasm of deprivation
stings panic into my lungs
And my body sinks deeper into
an untamable scream

I feel a tiny hand
the size of a baby starfish
tickle my belly
And a small voice murmur

"Just trust me, Mama."

And a current of faith
begins to undulate my fear to rest

And my body eases to the surface
And the sun kisses the top of my hair
And my face breaks the water's skin
And my lungs fill with life

And I let myself believe in him
In the possibility that is expanding
with each day inside my womb

He is spreading his hands
and kicking his feet
and turning his body

And he is giving me these words
to guide my synapses
to spark my wonder
and describe these sensations
and taste this beauty
and shape this color of my need

This life growing inside me
has a vocabulary all his own
Filled with phrases he learned from his angel brother

He is spelling out hope
with his fingers
and skin
and eyes
and limbs
and organs
Knitting their lives together

My body is creating
the second greatest poem
I will ever write

With all the words
I just learned to say
were theirs

December 13, 2006
9:23 a.m.

Quinn (brother of Avery) Adam Pullen was born
. . . and still lives

PART II

THE WAY FORWARD

CHAPTER TWENTY-TWO

Honoring and Remembering Your Baby

Janel C. Atlas

Birth is supposed to be the beginning of a lifetime of memory making. A squalling baby cries, a camera captures the first few hours, and the family meets its newest member. When the miracle of birth goes well, a bright future has begun. But for families whose babies die before they are born, birth is a milestone come too late. The dreams held close through the pregnancy (and for many expectant parents, for even longer than nine months) come crashing down, destroyed by the brutal, final hand of unexpected death.

But while stillbirth is an end, it is also a beginning: the start of a life as parents with one child forever missing. Mothers and fathers of stillborn babies often feel a powerful desire to hold that child's memory close as they explore how to remember the baby who will forever be a part of their family. Many parents' greatest fear is that their babies will be forgotten—that no one will say their babies' names. They worry that their babies died in vain, with no opportunity to positively touch others.

The concept of parenting your child's memory or parenting your child's legacy may be helpful. The energy that you would have devoted to caring for a newborn, teaching a toddler, and helping a young mind grow and develop need not stay dormant.

Many of the essays in this book reveal this deep desire to creatively channel energy into making meaning out of a baby's too-brief life. Some of the writers started foundations, organizations, or websites. Others started businesses, and still others counsel and support bereaved families through pregnancy and infant loss. Whatever path parents take to honor their child's life, practical actions of love can help the grieving process.

For the first year after my daughter's death, I had difficult days on the ninth of every month. It seemed like my subconscious was forever imprinted with the time of her birth (4:45 a.m.); I would wake up before dawn on the ninth, choked up and shaken. After this happened a couple months in a row, I learned to appreciate the way my system seemed to automatically know that I needed quiet days to cry and think about Beatrice. Thankfully, I had people who supported me and taught me to listen to my heart. They encouraged me not to act like everything was OK; instead, I marked the monthly date of Bea's birth on the calendar with a little star, in order to remind myself to make space and time to remember my precious baby. It was a small thing that enabled me to remember to have patience with my grief.

Some painful times are somewhat foreseeable, like your baby's birthday, the original due date, and so on. But sometimes the moments that swing parents into the depths of sadness are the little things: seeing another baby, smelling a certain scent that reminds you of the pregnancy or birth, watching a baby commercial, walking down the diaper aisle in the grocery store, hearing your baby's name, or even a gentle hug from a friend. Losing a baby isn't just a one-time loss; the pain reverberates in many ways and through the months and years of life beyond your baby's death, as the essays in part I explore.

While there is a natural ebb and flow to grief, there are also techniques you can use to make your way through the loss and life after. Like they helped the writers in this book, these methods can help you find ways to honor your child's legacy. These can take many forms and are as individual as each baby lost. Here are some ideas to get you started on this lifelong journey of honoring and remembering your baby. Not all of these will work for you, so feel free to select those that resonate with your personal experience and interests.

Mementos, Memories, and Ceremonies

Anything you have from your pregnancy, labor, delivery, and the weeks after can go in a collection of memories, stories, and ceremonies. Include anything that reminds you of your pregnancy and your baby, as well as anything that happened at birth and afterward. Cherish these things, as they will bring you comfort over time. You can keep making more to add to your basket of love, and pull out this collection whenever you need it.

Even if you came home from the hospital without any physical mementos from your baby's life and death, you can collect meaningful objects. For example, you can write a letter to your baby, save a program from a community memorial service you attend, sew a quilt, frame an ultrasound photo, and save condolence cards.

For me, ginkgo leaves will always remind me of Beatrice, because her cremains are buried under a ginkgo tree in the corner of my parents' property. Friends of ours generously gave me a beautiful ginkgo leaf pendant in memory of Bea; I love that I can wear it and know its significance without having to explain it to anyone. Many parents design tattoos in memory of their babies; drawing one alone or with the help of an artist can make a lifelong, meaningful illustration of your baby's presence in your life.

Other items you can include are poems (by you or by someone else), a collection of lullabies you sang to your baby, an outfit that you planned to dress your baby in, journal entries and photos from the pregnancy or the time after your baby's birth, and so on. Special jewelry, candles, seashells, stones, carvings, ornaments, art, books, and music can be gathered and held in memory of your stillborn baby. This can continue as the years go by; some parents buy or make items each year for a birthday or holiday.

A memorial box can be simple or ornate. At the memorial service we held for Beatrice, we asked those who wished to do so to write a letter (or draw a picture, if they were too young to write), which we then collected and put in our memory box. Some family members placed small items from their own childhoods in the memory box. I don't open the box often, but when I do, waves of gratitude and love flow through me as I see the many people who mourn Beatrice's death with me.

Whether or not you chose to hold a memorial service for your stillborn baby, you might want to participate at a public memorial service. Many hospitals offer a community time for remembering babies who have died. These services are often held in October, Pregnancy and Infant Loss Remembrance Month. Some cities have an annual Walk to Remember, as well. Other communities offer simple candlelit vigils; parents often express gratitude for the chance to remember their baby while being surrounded, supported, and validated by other families who understand how much life has changed.

Suz Pullen (chapter 21) created an altar memorial space in her home after her son's death. "In the months after Avery died, I was comforted by seeing reminders of him in a prominent place in my home—a place of honor. A place where I saw him and remembered that he had been real." A space for your baby's altar/memorial can be anywhere, like on the mantel or in the garden.

Just make sure, if you have pets or small children, that it's protected from accidental harm.

Holidays

Holidays often take on new meanings after the death of a baby. The calendar year and associative seasons will probably affect your grieving. As Laura Villmer's story (chapter 14) about her daughter's birth on Christmas Day shows, it's inevitable that family traditions and celebrations will be impacted by a death in the family. Just as an older loved one's death would require acknowledgment and a special tenderness the first spring, winter holiday, birthday, and death anniversary, the death of a baby before birth also impacts all those who love him or her.

There are many ways to incorporate the memory of a stillborn baby into family holidays. Give a gift in honor of your baby to a needy child. Place a special ornament or decoration that has your baby's name on it in a place of honor. Include your child's name on a family newsletter or in a card. Make a donation to a favorite charity in your baby's memory. Send out a note to family and friends reflecting on the grief and growth you've experienced since your baby was born. Give ample opportunity for surviving siblings, partners, grandparents, and others to share their memories, love, and grief, as well. When opening up the time and space to listen to other family members talk about their memories of the baby, you may receive some beautiful gifts. The death of a baby impacts the entire family system, so it makes sense that some of the healing may occur in community with each other.

Anniversaries

As the one-year anniversary of Beatrice's death approached, I felt stricken with fear that it would be horrible. I felt a sense of impending depression, and I worried that the day itself would pass in a slow, painful reliving of the day she was born. For me, the anticipation of the one-year anniversary of Beatrice's birth was significantly worse than the day itself. It helped that our family had decided to remember Beatrice with a trip to a lovely nearby park, and the release of a red balloon.

As Sherokee Ilse wrote (chapter 11), bereaved parents further along in the grief process often make plans for the anniversary/birthday, giving them more control and something special to anticipate, rather than to dread. Whether you find comfort in doing the same thing each year or in being open to whatever you feel led to do from year to year, give yourself permission to grieve your baby.

Traditions

Nearly all families whose children have died make their own traditions. The root of the word *tradition* is *traditio*, which means "handing over, passing on," as from one generation to the next. However, it helps me to think of tradition's root as also a means of relinquishing or releasing the pain associated with my dead daughter; implicit in the word is a recognition that life is fleeting and that there is tremendous value in passing on the lessons and values we hold close. In a way, by incorporating traditions into our family's life, my husband and I are trying to provide our living children with lessons hard-won through grieving our dead daughter: the ability to speak comfortably of someone who has died, a worldview that does not take tomorrow for granted because life is short, and the recognition that a loved one who dies is not forever gone from our family or memory.

The means of creating new family traditions vary by culture, religious background/spiritual beliefs, and many other factors. Give yourself permission to discontinue long-standing traditions if they are too painful. The healing aspects of ritual are well documented, and rituals need not be fancy or complicated. Anybody can develop a new ritual, and they can be celebrated alone or in a group. Here are some ideas for traditions others have found helpful. Pick and choose those that feel meaningful and authentic to you.

Write Your Own Story

Self-expression may be the primary purpose of writing your baby's story, but for those who are willing, blogs, websites, journals, scrapbooks, and essays can also increase awareness about stillbirth. Keep a journal or diary. Put your story to music. If you write about your personal experience and then find a way to share it, your words may reach out to others going through similar losses. As Kara L. C. Jones wrote in "Grief and Creativity" (chapter 20), "Amid the chaos, there was only one safe and sacred space I could go to express what was happening for me in any given moment: creativity." There are no judges, no censors, no one standing in disapproval. It's just you and a computer or a pen, and there's a freedom in committing your story to words.

Art

No matter what type of creative techniques you enjoy—quilting, knitting, cross-stitch, painting, jewelry making, sketching, sculpture, pottery—you can use it as a therapeutic and generous way to memorialize your baby. Even if you don't consider yourself to be a talented artist, using your hands to make something new can be a healing expression of love for your baby.

If you want to, try to find a way to donate your handiwork—to a silent auction for charity, to a medical center or hospital, et cetera. Check with the organizer to ask if you can attach a tag or note stating your baby's name and birthdate, or some other message in memory of your baby. By making a donation of something you created because of love for your baby, a small symbol of that love goes out and can encourage and help others.

And don't forget that what you find comfort in doing may speak to other bereaved parents as well. Parents of stillborn babies have started nonprofits and businesses making pregnancy and infant-loss jewelry, art, greeting cards, and websites.

Support a Cause

In the aftermath of your baby's death, did an institution or organization provide you with comfort? If you choose to offer your time or a financial contribution, you can help them continue their work. For instance, national groups like SHARE, First Candle, the March of Dimes, and the MISS Foundation rely on donations in order to reach out to people who need information and support. Threads of Love and Angel Layettes are two other organizations that rely on donations, which are then used to create beautiful blankets, gowns, and outfits that are donated to hospitals around the country.

Maybe there was a specific book that helped you; consider buying copies in bulk and donating them in your baby's name to hospitals, funeral homes, and libraries. If there isn't an advocacy/awareness group specifically about what caused your baby's death, perhaps you can start one in your area.

Don't forget to share information about these causes with family and friends. Someone you know may want to pitch in, too.

Volunteer and Perform Acts of Service

If you have a cause you care about, volunteer in your child's memory. Organizations are always looking for reliable volunteers, so follow your interests to help others. The work you do need not have a direct connection to the cause of your baby's death. For example, you can put loving energy into your local food bank, nursing home, or animal shelter.

Don't want to volunteer regularly, but still want to serve others? The MISS Foundation offers Kindness Cards (www.missfoundation.org/kindness/index.html) that you can print out and leave behind when you do an act of kindness. Here are a few suggestions for simple acts of kindness from Joanne Cacciatore, founder of the MISS Foundation:

- Buy a meal for a couple or family sitting next to you at a restaurant. Leave a Kindness Card with the waitress to give them after you leave.
- Buy shoes or clothes for a family in need.
- Bake cookies for a neighbor or teacher, just because.
- Help an elderly person with yard work or grocery shopping.
- Leave a bouquet at another child's grave at the cemetery.
- Find out if your electric company welcomes donations to help families who are struggling to pay their electric bills. Send in a payment with a Kindness Card.
- Bake goodies and take them to a police station, fire station, or hospital.
- Plug someone's parking meter.
- Adopt a street or just pick up litter in the neighborhood.
- Send your child a note in his lunchbox. Remind him how special he is to you.
- Look for opportunities to open the door for someone or give up your seat for someone.

When your heart is aching and your arms are empty, it is sometimes hard to look outside of yourself to see the needs of others. However, in performing small acts of generosity and love, we can elevate ourselves above the pain, even if only for a moment, to see life through someone else's eyes. In these small acts of kindness, we extend ourselves in service to others while simultaneously remembering our babies.

Support Others

Perhaps one of the most rewarding (yet difficult) ways to keep your baby's memory alive is to continue to tell your story at support groups and through other means, such as social networking sites, in websites, or even in letters to the editor. As Amy Abbey so clearly illustrated in her essay (chapter 18), parents who have experienced a stillbirth can help others by going to support groups to serve as a resource and encouragement for recently bereaved parents.

Inquire at local hospitals and birth centers to find out if there are other ways you can help support newly bereaved families, such as becoming a peer support parent or companion who can help them at the time of their loss or shortly after. Even if you do not do this in a formal way, consider going to meetings on occasion to share your story and listen in support as others share.

Also, be prepared for the moments when mentioning your child's name brings tears to an acquaintance's eyes, and you suddenly are the one comforting another bereaved parent. The compassion you have gained on the difficult grief journey of having a stillborn baby can truly bless others. You know firsthand what it is like, so you're probably the right person to reach out to others who are hurting.

If you aren't comfortable speaking up in a group or sharing your story with people in person, consider visiting or joining an online support community.

Unanticipated Grief

Parents whose babies died many years ago say that five, ten, or twenty years after the death, the grief still wells up, unexpected and unsolicited. There will be moments when you are going on with your life, making progress in a new normal, and a wave of sadness will suddenly crash over you. Sometimes your heart will feel just as broken as it did in the hours, days, and months after your baby died. The tears come without words and remind baby-loss parents that no one ever really *gets over* a baby's death. In those times of renewed pain about your baby, the tears can serve as a bittersweet reminder of just how much our babies taught us about love and loving.

While not all parents will feel the need to do things to honor and memorialize their babies, many, many parents do. The important thing is to find actions and ways of memorializing your baby that are meaningful to you. Even if no one else knows why you are doing the action, a great deal of joy comes from honoring a baby's life. Long after a baby has died, doing something as simple as spending a few moments in silence or performing an act of kindness in your child's memory recognizes the importance of one little life.

CHAPTER TWENTY-THREE

Creative Expressions of Grief

Kara L. C. Jones

Practical Aspects of Finding Your Own Creative Way

When grief comes, the last thing we feel is playful. Yet, in the face of this totally foreign landscape, we can choose to play out different options for finding our way, for choosing every creative moment. Given that there is no single answer to creatively addressing grief, I cannot say what choices will work for you. But I can offer a few suggestions on how you might begin finding your own creative way. You can try these on your own, in small groups, or in partnership with a coach or therapist.

Scribble to Self-Assess (Inspired by Cathy Malchiodi's *Art Therapy Sourcebook*)

Often we are so subject to what is happening to us, it is difficult to see through the chaos of grief. Instead of trying to escape the chaos, you can use the act of scribbling to lean into it instead. Here's how:

- Ask yourself what color your grief feels like today and get a marker, crayon, or chalk pastel of that color.
- Get a large piece of paper on which to scribble. You may want to put a larger piece of butcher paper underneath, so you can really flow with the scribble and not worry about going off the page.
- Close your eyes and with your nondominant hand, scribble out how the grief feels today. Let your hand just flow, round and round or back

and forth, but just keep your hand moving and scribbling. Do this till you feel done.

- Then open your eyes and look at the page. Turn it sideways and upside down. Look where the lines intersect and cross. See if any shape or image emerges to you. Take the time to enhance anything that emerges.
- Look also at the blank spaces between the scribbled lines. Do they say anything to you? Maybe consider filling them in with other colors. Or maybe words emerge that you want to write into the spaces. Work with the scribble until it feels done.
- You can try this several days in a row. Then hang them all up together and look at them as a storyline. See how your story shifts and changes day to day. See if there is anything surprising coming to the surface of the images. This can be a great alternative or supplement to writing in a journal.

Fill-In Poetry (Inspired by Poetry Workshop with Tony Curtis)

When looking at a blank page, it can be difficult to find the words to begin expressing your grief. Even if you are given a topic, like "Tell us how you feel today," it can be hard to face the blank page and come up with something touching on your actual experience in the moment. So we can take a sideways look at writing and find another way into sharing our experience on the page. Here's how:

- Take a look at the following prompts. Write them down or type them one by one and fill in your answer to each as you go:
    - *Today, my grief sounds like . . .*
    - *In my dreams, I had hoped to . . .*
    - *But when I look at my grief upside down, I see . . .*
    - *And on a bad day, my grief tastes like . . .*
    - *The three things I've learned . . .*
    - *With one eye closed, I see now that . . .*
    - *When I walk down the street, I . . .*
    - *And, today, my grief sounds like . . .*
- After you have finished filling in all your answers, read it all out loud as one piece of writing, as if it were one poem.
- When you are done, write and fill in at the top, as a title: "*Grief and the . . .*"
- Again, you can try this several days in a row, using it as a way to reflect on your experiences moving through the grief experience.

Body Tracing (Inspired by Beverly Naidus's *Arts for Change: Teaching Outside the Frame*)

In language and experience, we carry our grief with us in our bodies: "My heart aches." "I am wrestling with grief." "The news of her death knocked me off my feet." While we are probably not literally experiencing these things, we are using our bodies as metaphor. So for this exercise, we are going to more consciously begin using the shape of the body to express our grief. Here's how:

- Get three large sheets of butcher paper or art paper, big enough to lie down on and trace your body shape. You might want to get someone to do the tracing for you.
    - o On the first paper, write at the top, "The Moment of Trauma."
    - o On the second paper, write at the top, "When I feel unsafe in grief . . ."
    - o On the third paper, write at the top, "When I feel safe . . ."
- Then consider each of the body traces with those themes in mind. Look at the areas of the head, heart, stomach, hands, feet, reproductive organs, each in turn. Consider how your body felt at the moment of trauma. With each area of the body ask: Where did you feel it? What color did it feel like? Did it have a shape? Did the feelings have words you can put to them? Fill in the first body trace with colors, scribbles, drawings, and words to address each of these questions. Consider how your body feels when you feel unsafe or unable to fully express your grief and fill in that trace. Consider how your body feels when you feel safe, protected, and/or powerful in your expressions of grief and fill in that trace.
- When done, step back and look at all three pieces together. Look at how your story has unfolded since the moment of trauma. Consciously notice and try to remember how your body feels when you are unsafe. In the future, if you notice that feeling again, you can use it as a sign to change the situation or shift the circumstances to lean more toward the safe version of the body trace. Likewise, notice and try to remember how your body feels safe, supported, and empowered. Try to foster more of those situations and experiences as you explore in the future.

CHAPTER TWENTY-FOUR

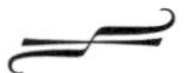

What We Know about Stillbirth

Ruth Fretts, MD, MPH

The terms *fetal death*, *fetal demise*, *stillbirth*, and *stillborn* all refer to the delivery of a fetus showing no signs of life. In the United States, there are significant variations from state to state about what types of loss are termed a stillbirth or fetal death. Many statisticians use the term *fetal death*, but parents prefer the term *stillbirth*—and slowly out of respect for parents, researchers are adopting this term. Of course, for parents with earlier losses, these are still babies who have died. It can be frustrating for parents to have their losses termed differently.

U.S. national data collect information on fetal deaths of babies 20 weeks of gestation or greater or, if the gestational age is unknown, babies that weigh 350 grams (about 12½ ounces) or more at birth. In the United States, there are many losses that are not included in the stillbirth statistics. Fetal losses related to terminations for lethal anomalies and stillbirths that occur during induced or augmented labors in pre-viable pregnancies (typically between 20 and 23 weeks) are specifically excluded from the stillbirth statistics; instead, these deaths are classified as terminations of pregnancy. This can be very troubling for parents. These definitions may seem arbitrary and somewhat punitive for a family who very much desired the pregnancy. What is called a stillbirth has been subject to much national and international debate.

In general, stillbirths can be subclassified according to the gestational age at delivery. *Early stillbirths* are typically defined as those occurring between 20 and 27 weeks of gestation, while *late stillbirths* occur at or after 28 weeks of gestation.

Frequency of Stillbirth

Within the United States in one year there are approximately 27,000 stillbirths.[1] The chance that a pregnancy will end in a stillbirth is 1/200 for white women and 1/76 for black women.[2] This is much greater than the number of infants who die after birth because they have chromosomal or congenital anomalies (5,600 per year) and those who die from Sudden Infant Death Syndrome, or SIDS (2,200 per year).[3] Worldwide there are an estimated three to four million stillbirths each year.[4]

In 2004, the stillbirth rate in the United States was 6.20 per 1,000 births, down from 6.41 per 1,000 in 2002.[5] Since 1990, the rate of early fetal loss (20–27 weeks of gestation) has remained stable at about 3.2 per 1,000, while the rate of late fetal loss (greater than or equal to 28 weeks of gestation) declined from 4.30 to 3.09 per 1,000.[6]

It is important to note that in the United States, black women have a rate of stillbirth twice the rate compared to that experienced by women of other ethnic groups. Asian, Native American, Hispanic, and white women all have stillbirth rates of less than 6 per 1,000 births, but black women have a rate of 11.25 per 1,000.[7] While black women appear to be at an increased risk of stillbirth throughout gestation, they suffer a greater proportion of losses between 20 and 24 weeks, as well as late losses (after 39 weeks of gestation). In fact, the rate of stillbirth for black women is 70 percent higher than for white women at 41 weeks of gestation, but black women are less likely to have their labor induced.[8] The reason for this increased risk of late stillbirth in black women is not known; some possible explanations include lack of societal awareness about this increased risk of stillbirth for black mothers, lack of access to quality medical care, underlying medical risk factors, and maternal stress.

General Causes of Stillbirth

The most useful information about the specific causes of stillbirth comes from hospitals or regions that systematically evaluate, review, and classify stillbirths. Dr. Robert Usher, a Canadian neonatologist, was a pioneer in the evaluation and classification of specific causes of stillbirth. In the McGill Obstetrical Neonatal Database (Canada), autopsy was a common tool used, with between 80 percent and 98 percent of stillborns undergoing autopsy over the four decades of the study. From this and other studies, we know that the specific causes of stillbirth vary according to gestational age.

Between 24 and 27 weeks of gestation, the most common known causes of stillbirth were related to infection (19 percent), abruption (14 percent), or fetal anomalies (14 percent); the reason for 21 percent of the stillbirths is not known.[9] After 28 weeks of gestation, the most frequent types of stillbirths were those that were unexplained, related to fetal growth restriction, and premature separation of the placenta (placental abruption). The proportion of stillbirths at term that remain unexplained is 40 percent.

A fetal death that is unexplained by fetal, placental, maternal, or obstetric factors is the most frequent type of fetal demise, representing between 25 percent and 60 percent of all fetal deaths. Variation in the proportion defined as "unexplained" generally reflects whether a stillbirth underwent a thorough evaluation, whether babies who are small for gestational age are included in this group, and whether possible cord accidents are included in this category.

No Known Cause

The most *common* type of stillbirth is that which is unexplained by fetal, placental, obstetric, or maternal reasons, even after thorough evaluation. Most unexplained stillbirths occur after 36 weeks of gestation and could potentially be prevented if these pregnancies could be identified prior to the demise. Unfortunately, there are no prospective trials of otherwise low-risk women to guide us, only observational studies. Studies have identified some risk factors for unexplained stillbirth, including advanced maternal age, obesity, low socioeconomic status, and very small and very large babies.[10] There does appear to be an interaction with first birth and advanced maternal age that places older women having their first birth at a 3.6-fold increased risk of stillbirth over younger women.[11]

While there have been no formal studies to evaluate the optimal surveillance and management of late pregnancy in otherwise healthy older women, in our collaborative practice, we offer either induction at 39 weeks of gestation for women forty years of age or older or twice-weekly testing. Prior to the 39th week in older mothers, we are more liberal in assessing fetal growth, strongly reinforce the value of kick counting, and perform regular nonstress tests (twenty minutes of monitoring the fetal heart to look for signs of well-being or possible trouble). But since there are no strong and clear data on the risks and benefits of this approach, individual practice varies considerably based on the practitioner's assessment of risk.

Fetal Growth Restriction (FGR) and Placental Pathology

The second most common type of stillbirth occurs in babies that are small for gestational age, with the most severely affected (weighing in the 2.5 percentile or less) having a greater risk than those between the 2.5 percentile and the 10 percentile. There are many reasons a baby might be smaller than expected, including birth order (parity), mother's height and build, and infant's ethnicity. Using a customized fetal growth chart that takes into account maternal characteristics such as height and weight improves the identification of babies who are at an increased risk of stillbirth and generates fewer "alarms" in healthy but small babies.

Poor fetal growth is assumed to reflect poor function of the placenta or other obstructions to fetal and maternal blood flow. Common associations with fetal growth restriction are fetal chromosomal abnormalities, fetal infection, maternal smoking, significant maternal hypertensive disease (high blood pressure), maternal autoimmune diseases like systemic lupus, maternal obesity, and maternal diabetes. A history of a previous growth-restricted baby being born preterm (earlier than 32 weeks' gestation) increases the subsequent risk of stillbirth eightfold.[12]

If a baby is found to be small for gestational age, an evaluation of blood flow through the vein in the umbilical cord can indirectly assess the function of the placenta, and this can be useful for determining if a baby needs to be delivered prior to term. Unfortunately, most stillborn babies who are significantly growth restricted are identified as growth restricted only at the time of the stillbirth, so the diagnosis of fetal growth problems remains a significant obstetric challenge. (For emerging research about IUGR and monitoring, see chapter 25.)

Abruptio Placenta

Premature separation of the placenta is the third most common cause of stillbirth. Fatal abruption is more common in the preterm fetus and is strongly associated with placental problems and inflammation.[13] The rates of abruption appear to be increasing in the United States and elsewhere. Maternal drug use is the strongest association among the maternal risk factors, but there are other important risk factors, such as smoking, hypertension, and preeclampsia. Cessation of smoking and drug use are important strategies, and past drug use should be gathered as part of the obstetric history. Also, women who report second- and third-trimester bleeding need to be considered high risk and have appropriate fetal monitoring, including periodic assessments of fetal growth.

Cord Accidents

The study of cord accidents has been difficult because at the birth of a stillborn baby careful systematic evaluation of the cord is not usually carried out. We know that about one in three live babies is born with one or more cords wrapped around his or her neck. With a live baby this is considered an incidental finding, but it is difficult to determine in the setting of a stillbirth if cord pathology is the *cause* of the death or an incidental finding. As of yet, no major comprehensive study has been done to determine how often cord pathology is linked to stillbirth, but on average, 20 percent of stillbirths are attributed to cord accidents by physicians.[14] Until we know more, it is important that when a stillborn baby is delivered with the presence of a cord-related issue (for example, torsion, knotting, or entanglement), a thorough evaluation of baby, mother, placenta, and cord be conducted in order to determine if there were other factors or conditions that could have contributed to the stillbirth. In addition, a photograph should be taken just after birth so the location of the cord around the baby and/or the cord's appearance can be reviewed at a later time. In addition to taking a postmortem photo of the attached cord, it can also be helpful to obtain an ultrasound picture prior to the baby's delivery, which can help determine the cord placement and condition. (For what researchers are discovering about cord accidents, see chapter 25.)

Multiple Gestations

Over the past two decades, U.S. rates of twin pregnancies have more than doubled and higher-order multiples have increased six- to twelvefold.[15] The rising number of multiples is due to increased use of assisted reproductive technologies and an increasing proportion of older mothers. The stillbirth rate among multiples is fourfold higher than singletons (19.6 per 1,000 versus 4.7 per 1,000).[16] The higher rates are due both to complications specific to multiple pregnancies (such as twin-to-twin transfusion syndrome) and to increased risks of complications common to singletons and multiples, in particular fetal abnormalities and growth restriction. Triplet or higher numbers of gestations are at high risk for multiple complications, including preterm birth and the death of one or more of the babies. Among twin gestations, it is recommended that fetal growth be monitored periodically; even in uneventful twin pregnancies, delivery is recommended by 39 weeks because of late unanticipated stillbirths.[17] Higher-order multiples are associated with even higher rates of perinatal death. One important strategy to reduce stillbirth may be to reduce the number of embryos transferred during an induced reproductive cycle.

Chromosomal and Genetic Abnormalities

Most pregnancy losses related to an abnormal arrangement of chromosomes usually occur early in gestation (and are termed miscarriages). But an estimated 10–12 percent of stillborn babies have been found to have a chromosomal abnormality.[18] Countries that offer prenatal screening for chromosomal or congenital anomalies and provide access to pregnancy terminations end up with lower rates of stillbirth. This is because pregnancies that are terminated are not included in the stillbirth statistics; they do remain, however, significant losses for parents, and can have significant psychological impacts on women in particular. For women who elect to carry to term a baby with Down syndrome, the risk of stillbirth is higher than normal.

Infection

In developed countries, stillbirths attributed to infection occur mainly in the premature fetus, and this rate has not changed much over the past decades. A substantial proportion of these deaths are related to an infection that originates in the vagina and then ascends to include the uterine cavity and the baby. Risk factors for these types of losses are cervical incompetence and multiple gestations. Infection can occur late in pregnancy, although it is relatively rare. The most common pathogens are E. coli, human parvovirus 19, and group B strep (GBS). (For more on GBS prevention and awareness, see chapter 25.)

In an ideal setting, if there is fetal hazard such as infection, lymphokines (an inflammation protein) will usually initiate labor, thus "rescuing" the baby by birth. But the factors in the mother and baby that are responsible for the initiation of labor are not known. There is a proportion of "explained" stillbirths that are really caused by infection, but for some reason the mother's body did not mount the appropriate response to initiate labor.[19] Some researchers have evaluated the inflammation response in otherwise unexplained stillbirths and have found significant genetic variations that inhibit an appropriate inflammation response.[20] To date this information has not translated into practical advice for parents, except that when a baby is stillborn and infection may not appear to be the cause of death, it is still worth having both the baby and placenta examined because infection is more common than one might think.

Considerations in Timing a Subsequent Pregnancy

Each person will have an individual response to the thought of trying to conceive again after a stillbirth. Not all women will want to pursue another pregnancy; it is a complex decision that involves many factors: the physical and mental health and well-being of the mother and/or the couple, her age, her fertility, and reproductive experience.

If a woman with a loss plans a future pregnancy, it is advisable to talk with her provider before conceiving. The interval between the birth of a stillborn and the *initiation* of a subsequent pregnancy has a measurable impact on the obstetric outcome. Optimal outcomes (fewer preterm births and pregnancy problems) occur if the interval is about one year.[21] This also gives the mother an opportunity to focus on healing psychologically and physically. I remind my patients that the mother must be strong enough to manage the usual risks and challenges of the first trimester (such as early miscarriages and prenatal screening).

Many women will feel a strong urge to move forward as soon as possible, but parents who do so may face additional emotional stress when the expected birth date of the subsequent pregnancy lines up rather closely to the time a year before when their stillborn baby was born or due.

A major consideration is the couple's age and fertility. Women who are older and who have a shorter window of opportunity to conceive should be encouraged to wait at least six months.

Tests to Request Prior to a Subsequent Pregnancy

Your provider should review the medical records from your previous loss. Some practices do blood tests during a pregnancy. However, if the following tests have not been recently performed, ask your provider for them:

- TSH test, which checks how well your thyroid is working.
- Recent rubella titre. Rubella (also called German measles) is a virus for which most women have immunity because they have been vaccinated. However, occasionally women are not immune, and rubella can cause stillbirth.
- An antibody level for parvovirus 19 antibody. Parvovirus is another common childhood virus that can (rarely) cause fetal anemia if the mother contracts it while she is pregnant.
- If your stillborn baby was very small, you may want to have a few blood tests done, including a lupus anticoagulant test and an anticardiolipin antibody test.
- The role of the thrombophilia workup is unknown at present. These are inherited differences in clotting factors. While earlier research suggested an association between thrombophilia and stillbirth, recent research places this association into question. Still, if you have a personal or a family history of blood-clotting problems, an evaluation of clotting factors is indicated.[22]
- If you had gestational diabetes in your last pregnancy, ask for an early glucose challenge test to see how well you metabolize carbohydrates.

- If you do not have a history of having chickenpox in the past, you should be tested to see if you have varicella antibodies.

Risk of Recurrence

While the risk of having another stillbirth is significantly related to the factors in the death of the stillborn baby—including etiology, maternal race, gestational age, and fetal growth restriction—the overall risk can be increased twofold to tenfold in a subsequent pregnancy.[23]

Women who have had a preterm stillbirth in which the baby was very small for gestational age have a higher risk of recurrence than women who have an unexplained stillbirth near term or who have had a stillbirth related to a cord accident. For any woman who was diagnosed during a previous pregnancy with a baby measuring small for gestational age, serial ultrasounds tracking the baby's growth can help the provider determine when it is safe to deliver the baby, rather than having the baby remain in the mother.

When a mother has severe medical problems, such as long-standing diabetes or kidney problems, the recurrence risk will be moderate, and these women will need to work closely with a doctor who deals with high-risk pregnancies to discuss if this is a safe and manageable option. Some recurrence rates may be lower for other stillbirth factors like, for example, the risk of subsequent stillbirth following a stillbirth due to a chromosomal abnormality, which is estimated to be less than 1 percent.[24] Each situation, however, is unique. A thorough evaluation of the previous loss, when possible, can help formulate a plan for a mother considering getting pregnant again. Women with a previous stillbirth usually desire more monitoring, need more care and reassurance, and appreciate a fairly structured plan of care. A woman who does not feel comfortable with the plan of care her provider proposes should feel free to get a second or even a third opinion or consider switching providers.

Typically, the management in the subsequent pregnancy involves preconception care, screening for infections, and first-trimester and/or second-trimester screening for fetal chromosomal and structural abnormalities. After 28 weeks' gestation, fetal surveillance should be tailored to the patient's previous history and anxiety. This care usually involves periodic ultrasounds for fetal growth.[25] I also reinforce the role of fetal-movement counting after 28 weeks of gestation. In the setting where the subsequent pregnancy continues uneventfully, I usually offer induction around 39 weeks, but again, this is tailored to the needs of each patient. Earlier deliveries are usually performed for obstetric indications such as hypertension, non-reassuring fetal testing, concern for fetal growth, or for a complaint of persistent decreased fetal movement.

Some providers consider delivering their patients prior to 37 weeks even if the baby appears to be doing well. The concern with this approach is that even babies born at 36 or 37 weeks can have problems breathing, nursing, and maintaining their blood glucose and body temperature. While these problems may seem minor compared to a stillbirth, they do add additional stresses and should be avoided if the baby seems to be thriving in utero. Most providers try to use more frequent fetal monitoring and extend the time the baby is in the mother rather than risk an early delivery, but again, there is considerable variation in practice.

Strategies for Prevention

There are general strategies for obtaining an optimal pregnancy outcome and more specific strategies for keeping track of fetal well-being. Some of these factors are not within a woman's control, but there are some that can be mitigated.

Sometimes a stillbirth is like the tip of an iceberg; other adverse pregnancy outcomes such as preterm birth and low birth weight have in common some social, behavioral, and demographic characteristics. We know that both extremes of maternal age have an increased risk of stillbirth. In 2004 in the United States, girls less than fifteen years of age had a stillbirth risk of 10.9 per 1,000 births; between the ages of fifteen and nineteen the rate was 7.5 per 1,000. The lowest risk of stillbirth was seen in women aged twenty-five to twenty-nine (5.5 per 1,000). Women between thirty-five and thirty-nine years of age had a risk of 7.2 per 1,000 births; women forty to forty-four, 10.4 per 1,000; and for women forty-five years of age or older the risk was 14.2 per 1,000.[26] We know that women who have late or no prenatal care, who smoke or take drugs, or who have poor nutrition are more likely to have a less than optimal outcome. Other risk factors include having a previous preterm birth, a small-for-gestational-age baby, medical conditions such as diabetes or preeclampsia, pregnancies with multiples, and second- or third-trimester bleeding. Still, the majority of women facing these risks will go on to deliver healthy babies. The challenge for providers and patients alike is to recognize and manage these risk factors to optimize the obstetric outcome.

In the setting where a low-risk woman embarks on a pregnancy, the advice and information should be balanced, keeping in mind that most of these women will have a baby to bring home. Advice for these patients generally falls under the realm of common sense: keep appointments; avoid food-borne infections; perform thorough handwashing; and avoid alcohol, smoking, and too much caffeine. Still, women need to know when they *should* worry, and be alert to warning signs of problems, including bleeding, unusual vaginal discharge, feeling unwell, unusual abdominal or back pain, or a decrease in fetal movement.

Decreased Fetal Movement

An estimated 4–10 percent of women report decreased fetal movement after 28 weeks of gestation. While most of these women will go on to have healthy babies, women who report this problem are at an increased risk of adverse pregnancy outcome, including fetal growth restriction, preterm delivery, and stillbirth.[27]

Unfortunately, the use of fetal movement counting fell out of favor when a large trial published in the British medical journal *The Lancet* compared two groups of women. One received information on how to formally keep track of their baby's movement using a fetal movement chart. The other group received information that they would be included in a trial as a control group, and that the goal of the study was to evaluate if using a kick chart helped reduce stillbirth.[28]

Prior to the study, the risk of stillbirth was 4 per 1,000 in singleton pregnancies after 28 weeks, but during the study, the risk was only 2.8 per 1,000 in both groups. The conclusion from this paper was that formal kick counting with a kick chart could not be recommended. However, an alternative conclusion could be that providing information on the importance of kick counting (either with a chart or just with information) was associated with a 30 percent reduction in stillbirth. Since this study is now almost thirty years old, we have learned that you cannot truly randomize vigilance and knowledge. Both groups benefited from participating in a trial designed to reduce stillbirth.

Currently there is no standard of care for the management of decreased fetal movement in the United States, so there is considerable variation in both the counseling of women and the subsequent management of the complaint by providers. Studies report that more than 50 percent of women wait forty-eight hours or more before contacting their provider when they have concerns that the baby is not moving well.[29] Once a woman arrives at her health care provider's office to be evaluated for decreased fetal movement, what happens next also varies considerably. Most frequently, women are evaluated using a nonstress test (NST), which monitors the fetal heart for about twenty minutes. It is often performed by a nurse; frequently, the obstetric provider does not evaluate the mother.

While an NST is a reasonable first test to assess if the baby is in immediate jeopardy of dying, this evaluation alone falls short. The complaint of decreased fetal movement should trigger a thoughtful review of the pregnancy, an evaluation of the patient risk status, and an assessment to determine if there is an evolving problem.

A 2009 study found that 24 percent of women who presented with the complaint of decreased fetal movement had babies that were measuring small for gestational age; this risk factor was not detectable if an ultrasound for fetal well-being was not performed.[30] Many times we do not take the time to review the overall pregnancy and risk factors. In the same study, researchers found that when a woman reports decreased fetal movement, health care providers improved their ability to predict which pregnancies are at a higher risk for an adverse outcome when the visit included these assessments:

- A clinical assessment that includes taking a history of the woman's past medical and obstetric history, including the number of times a woman reports decreased fetal movement
- A clinical evaluation of the uterine size using a tape measure (which is a low-tech way to assess the baby's size)

To strengthen the argument that guidelines for managing this problem are needed, a Norwegian quality improvement study demonstrated a *30 percent* reduction in stillbirths after a program of increasing maternal awareness and provider guidelines was initiated.[31] In the course of the study, pregnant women were given uniform information on kick counting at their ultrasound at 18 weeks' gestation. In addition, guidelines for the evaluation of decreased fetal movement reinforced that an ultrasound should be included in the evaluation of the complaint. This strategy was not associated with an increase in maternal anxiety—an expressed worry of some care providers.[32]

From my experience, the optimal management of decreased fetal movement is the following:

1. Being educated about fetal movement. I usually start discussing fetal movement with my patients around 28 weeks. I ask each mother to be mindful of her baby's movements. Each mother will find that her baby is sometimes active and sometimes sleeping. Some women report that the baby is very active and therefore think they don't need to formally count the movements, but I still review a counting strategy and report what is normal and what to do if they are concerned. I ask them to pick a time during the day when the baby is normally active; once the baby "wakes up" and starts moving, keep track of how long it takes the baby to move ten times. Typically it will only take about twenty minutes to get ten movements. If it takes longer than two hours, this may be a problem and she should call the office to voice her

concerns. There are many counting "rules," but this one is efficient because if you start counting when the baby is asleep it will take longer. Many women who are busy during the day don't notice the fetal movement (because there are only so many bits of information any person can process). However, I still reinforce the idea of keeping track of the fetal movement because an active baby is a healthy baby. As the baby gets closer to term, the sleep and wake cycles may get longer, and there may be less room to move—*but we still expect the baby to easily make the target of ten movements within two hours*.

2. Understanding what constitutes decreased fetal movement. If a woman is concerned that there is a significant decrease or absence of fetal movement, she should call her provider. Of course, this assumes that the woman has been consciously keeping track of the fetal movement, either formally using a kick chart or informally making mental notes to herself. There are some women who forgot to keep track during the day, and then when they lie down at night they think back on the day and grow concerned about the baby's movement. This is not the best way to keep track, because the baby may be sleeping. Some people will recommend eating something and lying down quietly to count fetal movements; if after two hours there are still concerns, she should go to the hospital for evaluation. Again, this advice should be tailored to the patient's risk factors and the patient's concern. However, I never recommend waiting until the morning if the mother is concerned that there is a decrease in fetal movements.

3. Requesting a thorough evaluation. When the patient is evaluated, the nurses and provider need to be on the lookout for problems, take a thorough history, assess blood pressure, and informally assess the fetal size by measuring the height of the uterus. The initial evaluation should include a nonstress test. Even if the woman reports that the baby is moving as usual and she feels reassured, I still follow up with an ultrasound within twenty-four hours. While the patient is there, I review kick counting, and tell the woman to call immediately if she has ongoing concerns about fetal movement.

4. Managing pregnancies with decreased fetal movement. If the patient is *preterm* (28–36 weeks), has been evaluated by her provider with both a nonstress test and an ultrasound, and no additional problems are detected, then fetal kick counting is continued. However, if there are additional concerns, the patient is encouraged to call the office for further investigation and evaluation. Sometimes an evaluation will detect potential problems like suspected growth restriction. In these cases, the pregnancies are monitored more closely, with ongoing evaluation of fetal growth and well-being.

5. Responding to decreased fetal movement at term. If the woman is overdue (past her due date by 1 week) and reports decreased fetal movement, I

offer induction. When the patient is at term or close to term, she will still be evaluated as above; the clinician is looking for potential problems. If the fetal testing (nonstress and ultrasound) are both normal but the patient complains of persistent decreased fetal movement in spite of the reassuring testing, I will discuss the option of inducing labor. Unfortunately, we do not know how often this strategy might avert a stillbirth or cause an unnecessary cesarean section. My view is that we should listen to mothers and babies. Very often, they are trying to tell us something.

Globally, the progress toward counting each birth and making each birth count has been achingly slow; this has been particularly true of stillbirths. In some ways, stillbirth is where SIDS was thirty years ago. Parents wanted to know why their babies died suddenly and silently in their cribs. They wanted answers, and some select researchers listened. The hard work of researchers, doctors, and advocates resulted in protocols for the evaluation of maternal and infant risk factors, autopsy protocol, and death scene analysis. Information from these studies culminated in the now widely followed recommendation to put babies "Back to Sleep." We now know that smoking is also an important risk factor for SIDS, and an education campaign has reduced the number of SIDS deaths by more than 60 percent. Now it's time to do the same research and hard work to find the causes and preventions for stillbirth.

Parents want to know why their babies died, and selected researchers are listening.

CHAPTER TWENTY-FIVE

Emerging Research

Janel C. Atlas

To find out about the cutting edge of stillbirth research and prevention, I spoke with some of the leading researchers and physicians around the world about the work they're doing. These are some of the experts I spoke with:

- Dr. Jason Collins, MD, cofounder of the Pregnancy Institute, is a practitioner who has worked with thousands of pregnant moms who have had stillbirths. For the past three decades he has studied the cord, its pathology, and the role it plays in stillbirth. Dr. Collins has been published in *The Placenta: Basic Science and Clinical Practice* and *Journal of the Louisiana State Medical Society*. As one of the tools to help prevent stillbirth, Dr. Collins uses an FDA-approved hospital-grade home monitoring device to detect problems with the baby during maternal sleep in pregnancies where the mother has had a previous stillbirth. This tool, combined with appropriate intervention at the hospital, has saved babies from stillbirth through early delivery when necessary. His site is www.preginst.com.
- Dr. Junichi Hasegawa, MD, PhD, is an obstetrician at Showa University Medical School in Tokyo. Dr. Hasegawa's work to prevent stillbirth has been published in the *Journal of Perinatal Medicine*, *Fetal Diagnosis and Therapy*, and the *International Journal of Gynecology and Obstetrics*.
- Jane Warland, RN, RM, PhD, Grad Cert Ed, is a lecturer in nursing and midwifery at the University of South Australia. Following the unexplained stillbirth of her daughter Emma, she wrote three books. Her

PhD research investigated the link among low blood pressure, location of the placenta, and stillbirth.
- Dr. Jason Gardosi, MD, FRCOG, FRCSED, is the director of West Midlands Perinatal Institute, Birmingham, UK. Dr. Gardosi's research has been published in many peer-reviewed journals.
- Dr. Mana Parast, MD, PhD, is an assistant professor at the University of California, San Diego, School of Medicine. Dr. Parast's research has been published in journals including *Human Pathology* and the *Journal of Cellular Biology*.

Of course, the medical information here is not meant to replace the care of a physician, midwife, or maternal health practitioner. You should talk to your health care provider to discuss your case and to map out a plan for a subsequent pregnancy. The research and perspectives provided here are not meant to be a comprehensive coverage of all of the possible causes of stillbirth. While 50 percent of stillbirths are not attributed to a particular cause of death, it isn't necessarily because there *isn't* an identifiable cause of death. With so little research being done on stillbirth epidemiology until recently, we just don't know enough about stillbirth yet to accurately determine what the cause of death may be. In many of the cases of unknown causes of stillbirth, there is a cause waiting to be determined.

For those parents who still do not know what caused their baby's stillbirth and wish to understand more, and for those contemplating subsequent pregnancies, the lack of information can create even more uncertainty and anxiety. Many bereaved parents consult the Internet or other parents for relevant information, but often the latest medical research that is published in journals or is under way at academic institutions can take a while to filter down into the hands of parents eager to find answers. In this section I provide a sampling of the emerging research focusing on potential causes of stillbirth that have, until recently, not generated much research or study, but may be contributing to many stillbirths. The following information reflects the research and views of the cited researcher or practitioner; it may not be the view of all who work in the field, or even the view of all of the other experts cited in this section. The information in this chapter is intended to highlight emerging trends in causes and prevention of stillbirth, and provide readers with information that may increase awareness and aid in prevention.

Cord Accidents

The umbilical cord is the lifeline running from the mother to her baby. A healthy cord contains three vessels: one vein, carrying oxygen-rich blood to the baby; and two arteries, carrying deoxygenated blood and waste away from the baby back to the placenta. It should be ropey, not too long and not too short, and contain enough Wharton's jelly to keep it from folding back on itself or getting knotted.

Because of the vital role the umbilical cord plays in nurturing and sustaining a baby right up through birth, any pathologies with the structure could possibly cause major problems and even stillbirth.

According to Dr. Jason Collins of the Pregnancy Institute, umbilical cord accidents (UCAs) are associated with about 8,000 stillbirths a year in the United States.[1] It is estimated, based on published world literature, that about 20 percent of all stillbirths are UCA-related, and there is evidence that UCA can be implicated as the cause of death.[2] The prevalence of stillbirths due to cord accidents is important to establish because "there is a worldwide tendency for medical professionals to discount UCA and look for other causes of stillbirths," says Collins, who has been working for years specifically on diagnosing cord problems and preventing UCAs. Usually, though, autopsy findings do not support the position that infection, congenital anomalies, placental disease, or genetic disorders are at fault. Instead, these stillbirths are most likely due to UCAs.[3]

Patients likely to have babies die of umbilical cord accidents often notice common patterns of fetal behavior. These warning signs may include the following:

1. Decreased movement, particularly at night. Pregnancy Institute studies have shown that babies who die because of umbilical cord accidents usually die during maternal sleep.[4] The tendency to note extremes of fetal behavior between 12 midnight and 6 a.m. is common among study subjects. (See below for more information about maternal blood pressure dropping at night. The combination of low blood pressure during maternal sleep and a cord anomaly can cause stillbirth.)

2. Fetal hiccups are another common indicator of UCA.[5] Most babies hiccup in utero some of the time or occasionally. Normal hiccupping sessions last from ten to fifteen minutes; this is not anything to worry about. However, you should contact your doctor about hiccups lasting longer than fifteen minutes and occurring frequently. Hiccuping is a fetal reflex that may show that the baby is trying to avoid umbilical cord compression. As an adult, you blink your eye to remove a speck of dust from it. The baby, in hiccuping, is attempting to get off his or her blood supply: the umbilical cord. If a baby has more than three episodes in a twenty-four-hour period, an ultrasound should be done to identify a possible umbilical cord problem. Cords and cord pathology can be seen on most ultrasounds.[6]

3. Collins reports that the women in his studies often describe babies with umbilical cord problems making "large arching movements, quivering, and performing sudden strong kicks."[7] In the only way they can, these babies are indicating their discomfort, as well as exhibiting reflex-driven attempts to maneuver into a better position. If a mother notices this behavior, she should ask for an ultrasound evaluation.

4. Another warning sign of a possible umbilical cord problem is if the baby's movement changes and he or she is unusually hyperactive (extreme movements) or hypoactive (less active than expected). If the mother notices this, she should go to a Labor and Delivery unit for a fetal evaluation. This evaluation should include a period of time during which the baby's heart rate is monitored to watch for decelerations (lower heart rate after the baby moves).

Noticing and recording fetal behavior (after 28 weeks' gestation) is a useful and relatively simple method to monitor the baby's well-being. A simple yet profound thing mothers can do to monitor their babies' health is to count kicks. The original kick-count method, created by Dr. E. Sadovsky, required mothers to note ten kicks in two hours.[8] Women whose babies are not active enough during this window of time should contact their medical care providers to check the baby (see chapter 24 for more information on kick-counting initiatives and guidance).

"Contrary to popular claims, umbilical cord problems are not random, and can often be predicted by knowing how to look for patterns," says Collins. "This information can empower mothers and their care providers to take steps that can help prevent an outcome of stillbirth." The clinical signs mentioned above—hiccups, changes in baby movement, and altered baby behavior—can warn a mother and her physicians that the baby may be in difficulty. The mother should have weekly prenatal visits if an ultrasound reveals cord problems such as multiple loops wrapped around the baby's neck (called a nuchal cord), true knots, or velamentous insertion of the cord into the placenta (in which the cord, instead of inserting itself into the middle of the placenta, inserts into the uterine membranes, then travels within the membranes to the placenta; the exposed vessels are not protected and are vulnerable to rupture). Babies with cord problems should be watched carefully and have frequent fetal heart rate recordings, called nonstress tests (NSTs). It is important to note that a cord accident does not usually kill the baby instantly; the baby may adjust to fluctuating blood flow through the umbilical cord and only succumb after several hours or days when he or she can no longer survive.[9]

Collins says that umbilical cord compression will always be obvious on an NST: "Any NST that shows a fetal heart rate declining to ninety beats per minute for one minute indicates that the mother needs to be admitted to the hospital for continuous monitoring."

It is now possible to identify more than forty different umbilical cord pathologies with ultrasound.[10] The detection rate of umbilical cord abnormalities is steadily increasing with the improvement of ultrasound technology. Because of these advances, the presence of an umbilical cord anomaly is an *identifiable* obstetrical condition that can be noticed based on clinical signs. With proper management, Dr. Collins believes that most babies with umbilical cord problems need not be stillborn.

In his practice in Japan, Dr. Junichi Hasegawa has implemented the practice of performing an ultrasound assessment of each fetus's umbilical cord. No risk factors are necessary to receive this assessment; every pregnant woman who receives care at Showa University Hospital, Tokyo, is given an ultrasound. In the eight years in which the obstetrics department has performed these ultrasounds, Hasegawa reports that the hospital has been able to avoid all cord accidents due to umbilical cord abnormalities, such as velamentous cord insertion, hypercoiled cord, and multiple entanglement of the nuchal cord.

One of the most dangerous (though less common) umbilical cord abnormalities is vasa previa. Vasa previa is when the umbilical cord attaches to the uterine membranes instead of to the placenta and the insertion point is below the baby's body in the uterus. These fetal vessels are easily compressed or ruptured when uterine contractions or membrane rupture occurs, resulting in fetal blood loss. While the incidence of vasa previa is very rare, estimated at about 1 in 1,200 to 1 in 5,000 pregnancies,[11] in the cases not prenatally diagnosed, the survival rate is only 50 percent. Diagnosis of vasa previa before birth with ultrasound and elective cesarean section would reduce the high fetal mortality rate due to vasa previa.

Velamentous cord insertion is often associated with preterm delivery, abnormal fetal heart rate pattern, emergency cesarean section, poor neonatal outcomes, and stillbirth. Unfortunately, there is nothing that can be done by either a woman or her physician to prevent these cord problems from occurring. What physicians can do, however, is make concerted attempts to find these abnormalities by precise ultrasound scan during the second trimester, then offer frequent observation and careful management of the birth, which might include an early delivery.

Multiple nuchal cord entanglements (more than twice) and extremely hypercoiled cord are also associated with perinatal complications. Third trimester ultrasounds are used to detect these problems. For most serious cord problems (other than vasa previa), strictly conducted *planned* delivery should be chosen. The hospital should use continuous fetal heart rate monitoring during labor or induction of labor. Fetal heart rate abnormalities during labor, such as tachycardia (fetal heart rate too fast) or bradycardia (fetal heart rate too slow), will indicate if the baby is in distress, and immediate action can be taken for safe delivery.

Since it's impossible to prevent such cord abnormalities from forming during pregnancy, Hasegawa recommends that every obstetrician work to detect such abnormalities before delivery at a prelabor checkup.

Recurrence of Cord Accidents

Answering the question about the risk of having another cord accident is difficult because there are only a limited number of controlled studies about this. However, some doctors have no doubt that umbilical cord accidents can and do recur in the same mom.[12] And according to the National Institute of Child Health and Human Development (NICHD), stillbirth can recur with a risk of five times the normal chance.[13]

In a case study of twenty-five women with a previous stillbirth, Collins interviewed the patients about their pregnancy losses and apparent causes. Patients were then offered an evaluation at between 28 and 30 weeks' gestation; the visit consisted of a thirty-minute fetal heart rate recording and an ultrasound for UCA recurrence. Mothers were then instructed on home use of a hospital-grade fetal monitor. Patients were monitored for thirty minutes every night, with recordings sent via the Internet to Collins at the Pregnancy Institute.[14]

Out of the twenty-five patients, twenty-one had UCA recurrence at 28 to 30 weeks' gestation. Fourteen patients delivered with a recurrent UCA, and all of the patients delivered by 37 weeks. Two patients had expedited C-sections for fetal heart rate decelerations during labor. No recurrent stillbirths occurred.

Because it appears as though umbilical cord problems can recur in subsequent pregnancies—though further research is needed to more fully understand how high the risk is—it is important to pay special attention to patients who have had a stillbirth.[15]

Patients with histories of stillbirth due to cord accidents should be considered high-priority patients, meaning that, while not every baby is at risk of dying, some may die if their medical providers do not manage them carefully. This priority status means these patients need more attention, more nonstress tests (NSTs), and more ultrasounds. The baby should be delivered no later than the due date—if not before—if there is any question of his or her well-being.

Low Blood Pressure

Throughout a pregnancy, an obstetrician or midwife measures a pregnant woman's blood pressure. Maternity health care providers have known for a long time the serious risks associated with high blood pressure (hypertension) during pregnancy. Blood pressure is considered high in pregnancy if the lower reading—called the diastolic reading—is consistently above 90.

Because doctors have long focused concern on diagnosing and treating high blood pressure, there is no standard definition of low blood pressure in pregnancy. Therefore, obstetric care providers currently consider anything less than 90 diastolic to be good. Although there have been a number of studies performed that have examined the impact of low blood pressure (hypotension) on poor pregnancy outcome such as bleeding from the placenta and small infant size,[16] until recently there has not been a study that specifically looked at the impact of low blood pressure on stillbirth (according to Jane Warland, who did her PhD research on hypotension and stillbirth).

Warland's PhD findings were reported in 2008.[17] She looked specifically at the incidence of low blood pressure in pregnancy and the risk of stillbirth. Blood pressure recordings from all prenatal visits of 124 women whose pregnancies ended in stillbirth were compared to blood pressure readings of 243 women who gave birth to living babies. The study found that women with a diastolic blood pressure reading between 60 and 70 mmHg throughout the pregnancy were about 1.5 times more likely to suffer a stillbirth. The study also found that if the diastolic reading was *always* less than 60 mmHg, the pregnant woman was 3.5 times more likely to have a stillbirth than those with higher diastolic readings. The most important number to record is the diastolic reading, as low systolic readings (the upper reading) do not appear to indicate an increased incidence of stillbirth.

Warland found that three mean arterial pressure (MAP) readings of less than 83 during the course of the pregnancy carried almost double the risk of stillbirth. MAP is calculated using the following formula:

$$\text{MAP} = [(2 \times \text{diastolic}) + \text{systolic}] / 3$$

You can use figure 25.1 to calculate your MAP. For example, if you have or had a systolic reading of 100 (on the top line of the chart) and diastolic reading of 70 (on the column on the left side), your MAP is 80. This is in the risky range. In contrast, a blood pressure reading of 120 over 80 results in a MAP of 93, which is not in the risky range.

Systolic Blood Pressure

Diastolic Blood Pressure	90	95	100	105	110	115	120	125	130
40	57	58	60	62	63	65	67	68	70
45	60	62	63	65	67	68	70	72	73
50	63	65	67	68	70	72	73	75	77
55	67	68	70	72	73	75	77	78	80
60	70	72	73	75	77	78	80	82	83
65	73	75	77	78	80	82	83	85	87
70	77	78	80	82	83	85	87	88	90
75	80	82	83	85	87	88	90	92	93
80	83	85	87	88	90	92	93	95	97
85	87	88	90	92	93	95	97	98	100
90	90	92	93	95	97	98	100	102	103
95	93	95	97	98	100	102	103	105	107

Key:

Extremely Low MAP	(hatched)
Borderline Low MAP	(gray)
Normal MAP	(white)
High MAP	(black)

Figure 25.1. Chart for Determining Mean Arterial Pressure (MAP). From J. Warland (2006).

So, why is low blood pressure related to an increased risk of stillbirth?

Warland's study found that women whose blood pressure falls in the borderline low range appear to be at higher risk of stillbirth than those in the extremely low group. This may be because the borderline group is subject to wider variation in blood pressure from daytime to nighttime. Maternal blood pressure—the force exerted by blood pushing against the arterial walls—directly influences the flow of blood to the placenta, and thus to the baby. If the mother's blood pressure is too high, the oxygen- and nutrient-laden blood rushes past the fine blood vessels in the placenta, depriving the baby of what he or she needs. If the mother's blood pressure is too low, says Warland, it's possible there isn't enough pressure for these placental vessels to get blood, and therefore oxygen and nutrients, to the baby.

Because blood pressure typically drops when you're asleep, if you have borderline low blood pressure readings during the day, your blood pressure might fall to extremely low levels during sleep. This may be one reason why some babies of mothers with hypotension die between midnight and 7 a.m.[18] It may be that there is a threshold level of lowest blood flow to the placenta, and if blood pressure falls below this level when the mother is sleeping, the baby can't survive.

Managing a Pregnancy with Low Blood Pressure

The very first step toward a positive pregnancy outcome is being aware that low blood pressure isn't always a good thing. It may be necessary for you to educate your health care provider by sharing this chapter with him or her. Usually doctors are open to reading new studies and learning about new methods to help their patients.

If your blood pressure were high, your health practitioner might prescribe a blood pressure medication. However, because of the well-documented negative effects of high blood pressure during pregnancy, no obstetric care provider will prescribe medication to raise your blood pressure. Therefore, it is vital that you be carefully monitored throughout your pregnancy and that you take steps to keep your baby safe.

One of the most important things you can do is to become attuned to the times your baby is active or asleep. If you notice that these times change, you should immediately see your health practitioner or midwife. Regular fetal monitoring through biophysical profiles and nonstress tests can give you some reassurance and provide your health care provider with helpful information about your baby's health.

Though most pregnant women know not to sleep on their backs, it is especially important for women with low blood pressure to avoid lying that way. Back sleeping is a concern because that position during pregnancy can cause a drop in blood pressure. If you already have low blood pressure and lie on your back, the possible drop in blood pressure might endanger your baby. If you sometimes wake up to discover that you've shifted onto your back in your sleep, position a small pillow or wedge to keep you from rolling onto your back. You may also consider wearing compression (also called antiembolic) stockings at night to prevent pooling of blood in the lower limbs and allow the maximum amount of blood flow to the placenta.

Placental Problems

The placenta, also known as the afterbirth, connects the baby to the wall of the womb in order to allow exchange of nutrients and waste. It implants in the lining of the uterus (womb), and a vast array of tiny blood vessels branch through it into the uterine wall. Blood flowing from the baby through the cord's arteries goes through the placenta, where it is carried very close to the mother's blood for the exchange of oxygen, nutrients, and antibodies. The blood then returns through the cord's vein, carrying with it the things the baby needs to grow and thrive.

Problems with the placenta that can cause stillbirth include the following:

1. *Placental insufficiency and failure*. When the placenta does not work efficiently, the baby does not get enough nutrients and/or oxygen to thrive. It can be difficult to diagnose placental insufficiency early in pregnancy, because even a placenta with problems can often provide enough sustenance to the baby until growth accelerates rapidly during the late second trimester and third trimester.[19]

2. *Placental infarction (tissue death)*. Often caused by preeclampsia or maternal hypertension, placental infarction occurs when a part of the placenta dies. Sometimes during an otherwise healthy pregnancy, a small section of the placenta may die off; as long as the remaining healthy part of the placenta can provide sufficient oxygen and nutrients to the baby, this will not cause stillbirth.

3. *Bleeding*. Bleeding during pregnancy is very scary, though it does happen often, usually in the first trimester. Any bleeding should be reported to your health care provider. Immediate medical attention may help determine the cause and reduce the chances of harm to the baby and mother. Hemorrhage is most often caused by placental abruption and placenta previa. Placental abruption occurs when the placenta, either in part or in whole, detaches from the uterine wall. The result depends on the level of separation. A woman whose placenta pulls away only a little bit may experience bleeding and some pain. Recommendations for these types of cases include complete bed rest and other means of preventing premature labor. However, in severe placental abruption, most or all of the placental membranes detach from the uterus, and the baby is cut off from his or her oxygen supply. In this type of obstetric emergency, doctors often perform an emergency C-section to try to save the baby's life, and the mother often may need a blood transfusion because of blood loss.

Placenta previa is a condition in which the placenta lies over all or part of the cervix. This can be diagnosed at the 20-week ultrasound. In many cases, this resolves itself as the uterus expands. However, a low-lying placenta as labor approaches can be dangerous, as the placenta can separate from the uterus as the cervix thins and opens.

Recent research has shown that women who have a posterior-located placenta—a placenta located on the back wall of the uterus—are 1.5 times more likely to suffer a stillbirth than women who have a placenta in an anterior (front) position.[20]

This is a relatively new finding, and more research is needed to determine exactly why this puts babies at an increased risk of being stillborn.

Dr. Jane Warland, the author of the study, says that there are three possible reasons:

1. The structure of the posterior uterine wall is somehow at fault. A placenta located on the posterior uterine wall may be somehow less efficient due to the anatomy of that wall. Blood supply to the uterus is not uniform,[21] and the posterior wall of the pregnant uterus is longer[22] and somewhat thicker.[23] Each of these factors may affect maternal blood supply, especially as the uterus expands to accommodate the pregnancy.

2. There are some other (as yet unknown) risk factors associated with a posterior-located placenta. A posterior-located placenta may be associated with increased risk of stillbirth because of other risk factors for stillbirths that are also linked with it—for example, nuchal cord (umbilical cord around the infant's neck). It may be that babies with both a nuchal cord and posterior-located placenta are at increased risk.[24]

3. Another possible reason that might explain why a posterior-located placenta is associated with an increased risk of stillbirth is maternal sleeping position. If a woman with a posterior placenta sleeps on her back, it is possible that the weight of the pregnant uterus overlying the placenta might compromise placental blood flow.

Of course, as with cord formation and structure, there is nothing you can do to move the position of the placenta. Simply being aware that this may put you at an increased risk of stillbirth can provide your health care provider with the information he or she needs to monitor your pregnancy more closely for possible problems.

Similar to cases of possible cord abnormalities, mothers with posterior placentas should take the time to notice and record their baby's movements and habits. If those habits change, see your health practitioner. Most providers would prefer an extra visit to the office for a quick heart rate check or nonstress test rather than miss a sign the baby isn't thriving.

Intrauterine Growth Restriction

Intrauterine growth restriction (IUGR), also known as fetal growth restriction (FGR), is the condition in which the baby in the womb fails to grow according to its own optimal growth potential.

There can be a number of causes, including congenital anomalies or infection early in pregnancy. However, the most common cause, responsible for over 80 percent of cases of IUGR, is that the placenta is not functioning well.[25] It is then unable to carry sufficient oxygen and nutrients from mother to baby. As a result, a baby whose growth has looked normal up to a certain point in the pregnancy may suddenly show a decline in growth. Often, the cause is the placenta not establishing itself well on the wall of the uterus early in pregnancy. Doctors are still trying to find the reason why this occurs.

According to Dr. Jason Gardosi, IUGR occurs in 10–20 percent of all pregnancies.[26] It has an increased chance of occurring when the mother smokes, takes drugs, or drinks excessive alcohol. Mothers over forty and those who are either very thin or obese have an increased risk of IUGR as well. Women with hypertension or preeclampsia also have an increased chance of IUGR. Social deprivation is also linked, although it is uncertain whether this is due to poor nutrition or other causes.[27]

IUGR is the single most common *clinical* cause of stillbirth: in about 40 percent of all stillbirths, the baby had IUGR before he or she died.[28] If lethal congenital abnormalities are excluded, over half of all normally formed stillborn babies had IUGR.

Customized Growth Charts

Until recently, most doctors and midwives used the same fetal growth chart for all their patients, even though it has been recognized for years that the mother's weight and height, her ethnic group, and the parity (birth order) of the pregnancy all play into determining the baby's size.

However, Gardosi and his team have pioneered the use of customized charts and made them freely available for download from the Internet (www.gestation.net). The charts are now in use in many units in the UK, Australia, and New Zealand, and they are being recommended in guidelines such as those from the Royal College of Obstetricians and Gynaecologists.[29] The charts are more effective in detecting babies who really are IUGR by comparing the actual growth of the baby against the optimal growth potential calculated for each mother in each pregnancy.[30]

"Customised charts improve the detection of the baby's growth, as determined by measurement of the fundus—the height of the womb—or ultrasound scan, to estimate the baby's weight," explains Gardosi. "The charts can also be reassuring for mothers and their midwives and doctors and reduce the need for unnecessary investigations."[31] For example, Gardosi explains, a 6½-pound estimated fetal weight might be a normal-sized baby for a small mom but might be IUGR for a bigger mom who should be expecting a much heavier baby.

As with placental and cord problems and maternal hypotension, good monitoring of the baby during the pregnancy is key to reducing the risk of stillbirth. For IUGR, growth during pregnancy requires sequential measurement of the womb (fundal height), plotting on customized charts, and referral for an ultrasound if the measurements do not follow the expected growth curve.[32] If the ultrasound suggests the baby is small, a Doppler measurement of blood flow through the umbilical cord will help in assessing how well the placenta and cord are functioning.[33]

Currently, the only treatment for IUGR is well-timed delivery. On a case-by-case basis, the practitioner must use all the gathered data to weigh the risk of delivering an at-risk baby early versus leaving it in the mother for too long, when the result might be stillbirth or other complications due to IUGR.

Mothers who have had a stillborn baby found to have been IUGR or who have had a live born baby with IUGR are most likely to have a normal outcome in their next pregnancy. However, the chance of recurrence is increased. Therefore, women with previous stillborn babies or live born babies with IUGR need to be monitored carefully with sequential ultrasounds to check that subsequent babies are growing well.

Infections

A pregnant woman comes in contact with many bacteria and viruses throughout the time she carries her child inside her uterus. Thankfully, many of those potentially dangerous infections do not infect the mother or are unable to pass through the placental barrier. However, certain infections can harm the developing baby.

Some of the organisms that can cause profound problems for the unborn baby are cytomegalovirus (CMV), human parvovirus B19 (Fifth Disease), listeriosis, rubella (German measles), and toxoplasmosis. These are called ascending infections, meaning they pass from the mother's body to the baby.

One bacterium about which scientists know a great deal is group B streptococcus (GBS). A common bacterium that naturally lives in the intestinal tract of one in four women, GBS poses a risk to babies in utero as well as after birth. GBS infections in newborns can lead to respiratory failure and pneumonia that can progress rapidly into a blood infection, septic shock, and death, according to Group B Strep International.[34]

Pregnant women in the United States and some other countries are screened for GBS bacteria between 35 and 37 weeks of pregnancy. If GBS is detected, these women are given intravenous antibiotics during labor to protect their baby from contracting the infection. The risk of GBS in healthy adult women is minimal.[35] The current methods of preventing the spread of GBS have met success in preventing early-onset infection between birth and one week old. However, the rates of GBS-related stillbirth, preterm birth, and late-onset infection (occurring in infants after the first week of life up to several months of age) are not decreased or prevented by the current prevention strategy.

Emerging GBS research includes utilizing molecular genetics to increase understanding of the disease-causing Gram-positive bacteria and continued efforts to develop a GBS vaccine.

How Do We Learn More?

In order for us to continue learning more about stillbirth causes and prevention, more attention must be given to improving data collection by promoting standardized, thorough reporting and recording of stillbirth data; conducting a large-scale comprehensive study of stillbirth; and encouraging the practice of performing thorough and well-documented autopsies.

Autopsy

First, standardized, thorough autopsies can be instrumental in determining a cause of death, but communicating the need for or benefits from autopsies to newly bereaved parents can be challenging for health care providers. For more information about autopsies, in particular what we can learn from them, I consulted Dr. Mana Parast.

While we usually think of an autopsy as a scientific examination of a body, when the deceased individual is a stillborn baby, it is vital for medical personnel to send the placenta and cord to pathology for careful examination, particularly in cases of third-trimester stillbirths.[36] Parast points out that this is because, while a significant subset of first- and early-second-trimester losses are due to health problems with the baby, the majority of late-second- and third-trimester losses have at least part of their origin in the placenta.[37] Therefore, a thorough visual examination of the placenta is very helpful, but the most detailed and conclusive autopsy exams include an autopsy of the baby's body, a visual exam of the placenta, and a microscopic exam of the placenta.

Problems that can arise from the placenta or compromise placental function include the following:

1. *Infection*. Many times, signs of infection are present in the placenta, but it is sometimes not possible to identify or culture the specific microorganism.

2. *Placental insufficiency*. The placenta supplies the growing baby with what he or she needs from the mother, so if the placenta undergoes changes related to hypertension and preeclampsia, it may not be able to provide enough oxygen and nutrients. In severe cases, placental insufficiency is associated with fetal growth restriction.

3. *Umbilical cord abnormalities*. As many otherwise healthy babies are born with cord abnormalities, specific findings from microscopic examination of the placenta help establish whether an umbilical cord accident is the cause of stillbirth.[38]

4. *Abruption*. Placental abruption is the separation of the placenta from the site of uterine implantation before delivery of the baby. While this can be caused by trauma such as a car accident, says Parast, the majority of placental abruptions are thought to be due to abnormal blood vessels in the uterine wall.

5. *Fetal-to-maternal hemorrhage*. This is caused by rupture of a fetal vessel in the placenta, and leads to fetal blood loss into the placenta. This diagnosis can be suspected on a placental examination but can only be confirmed by a maternal blood test (called the Kleihauer-Betke test).

In addition to the above specific findings, one of the most important pieces of information we can learn from microscopic examination of the placenta is *when* the stillbirth actually occurred, says Parast. Changes seen under the microscope in fetal vessels in the placenta can give a relatively accurate estimate of the time of fetal demise in utero.[39] This information puts other findings in the placenta or fetal autopsy in perspective by helping to distinguish premortem findings (potential causes of stillbirth) from postmortem artifact.

Stillbirth Reporting Protocol

Second, without a standardized stillbirth reporting protocol from hospital to hospital, county to county, and state to state, researchers will still be unable to understand the true scope of stillbirth. One joint effort is currently under way through the Iowa Stillbirth Surveillance Project and the Centers for Disease Control. They are creating a stillbirth registry that serves as a model for the rest of the nation.

The Iowa Stillbirth Surveillance Project was inspired by four Des Moines–area moms, each of whom lost a daughter to stillbirth in 2003. The group of moms, State Representative Janet Petersen, Jan Caruthers, Tiffan Yamen, and Kerry Biondi-Morlan, wanted to do something to ensure other parents wouldn't have to endure the heartache of losing a baby; they started a crusade to get people talking about stillbirth.

Their talks resulted in the idea of a stillbirth registry, which would serve as a central repository for the collection of consistent stillbirth data, including information about the baby as well as the mother's health and her pregnancy.

At the time, the reporting and management of stillbirth cases in Iowa, as throughout much of the United States and the developed world, was not consistent. Legislation creating a standardized registry was passed by the Iowa House and Senate and was signed into law by the governor in 2004.

The Iowa Stillbirth Surveillance Project was divided into two phases. In phase 1, the Iowa Department of Public Health convened a work group of experts to design a standardized fetal death evaluation tool. The makeup of the group ranged from obstetricians, perinatologists, and pathologists to grief counselors, insurance company representatives, and stillbirth parents. This group wrote a Stillbirth Evaluation Manual designed to help health care providers collect consistent demographic information, patient history/ patient interview, and pathology/postmortem reports, and provide information and resources for appropriate follow-up care and grief support. These manuals were disseminated to every birthing hospital in Iowa and to all Iowa physicians who practice obstetrics.

In phase 2, the Iowa Stillbirth Surveillance Project got assistance from the Centers for Disease Control and Prevention (CDC). As the recipient of a cooperative agreement with the CDC, the Stillbirth Surveillance Project conducted a pilot project to expand its existing birth defects state registry to include surveillance for all fetal deaths in Iowa.

Today, Iowa leads the nation in stillbirth data collection, and sets an example for other states and regions to strive for. Efforts are under way to build a national stillbirth registry.[40]

Controlled Study

Finally, a comprehensive controlled study of stillbirth across demographic populations is necessary in order for us to accurately investigate stillbirth occurrences and causes. Below, Catherine Y. Spong, MD; Uma Reddy, MD, MPH; and Marian Willinger, PhD, explain the Stillbirth Collaborative Research Network (SCRN):

> In 2000, the National Institute of Child Health and Human Development's (NICHD) Pregnancy and Perinatology Branch held a workshop on stillbirth to understand the state of knowledge and gaps. This meeting culminated in an executive summary and a series of publications in *Seminars in Perinatology* highlighting the presentations at the meeting (2001). The findings from this workshop highlighted the urgent need for more research given that stillbirth occurs in 1 in every 150–200 pregnancies in the U.S. At a rate equivalent to the infant mortality rate in the United States, stillbirth is a significant problem and over 50% of stillbirths remain unexplained. The NICHD established the Stillbirth Collaborative Research Network (SCRN) in 2003 to explore the epidemiology and causes of stillbirth.
>
> This network includes five clinical centers: Women and Infants in Providence, RI, The University of Texas Medical Branch in Galveston, Texas, the University of Texas in San Antonio, Emory University in Atlanta, GA, and

The University of Utah in Salt Lake City, Utah. The network includes an independent data center, the Research Triangle Institute in North Carolina and staff from NICHD. In total 59 hospitals from the five clinical sites participated to obtain a geographic population-based determination of the incidence of stillbirth. Stillbirth was defined as fetal death at 20 weeks of gestation or greater. The study also obtained information to determine the causes of stillbirth using a standard stillbirth postmortem protocol, to include review of clinical history, protocols for autopsies and pathologic examinations of the fetus and placenta, other postmortem tests to illuminate genetic, maternal, and other environmental influences and elucidate risk factors for stillbirth. Enrollment of 663 stillbirths and 1932 live births among 59 hospitals was completed between March 2006 and August 2008. This is the largest study of this topic in the United States and the largest case-control study worldwide.

Some preliminary results of this study were presented at the Society for Maternal Fetal Medicine meeting in January 2010 and the Society for Gynecologic Investigation in March 2010.[41] The causes of death were assigned using the information from a standardized research protocol, which included autopsy, placental pathology, maternal interview, medical record abstraction, and laboratory analyses. The majority of stillbirths, 90%, occurred before delivery (antepartum) and with a complete work-up, 60% were identified with a probable cause of death. The most common causes were placental insufficiency, obstetric complications, infection, maternal medical conditions, genetic/structural anomalies and cord abnormalities. Several demographic and pre-pregnancy risk factors were identified, including extremes in maternal age (age <20 or >39 years) and maternal weight (BMI <18.5 or >24.9), maternal race, stressful life events, prior stillbirth, maternal conditions (hypertension, diabetes), and smoking. Although no association was found between several thrombophilias (prothrombin gene, PAI-1 and MTHFR), there was an association between the factor V Leiden mutation and stillbirth.

This study is a rich resource for future research on various aspects of stillbirth. Information about the network and its findings are available at https://scrn.rti.org. This study will also provide valuable information on how best to determine the cause of death and therefore the management of subsequent pregnancies. As our understanding of the causes and risk factors for stillbirth improves through further research, potential interventions may be developed to prevent the occurrence of this devastating outcome.

Even with many devoted researchers around the world working on various questions about stillbirth, how and when it strikes, and means of prevention, stillbirth still claims about thirty thousand babies in the United States and four million worldwide each year. With the tools at our disposal, including preconception health, preconception genetic therapies, assisted fertility techniques, monitoring, testing, measuring, and labor/delivery tools and methods, too many babies are born without a chance to take a breath. Too many parents go home with empty arms and aching hearts, their months of waiting resulting in a silent nursery. But hopefully the work being done in these areas of emerging research can continue to help health care professionals and parents gain answers to the millennia-old question of why stillbirth happens. Perhaps with better understanding, enhanced diagnostic capabilities, and improved awareness, we will be able to dramatically diminish the risk of babies dying before they take their first breath.

Resources

Many of the organizations and groups listed here may provide more than one type of resource. We have listed them in one primary category, but we have listed the additional work they do. Many of these organizations have extensive information, resources, and links to other helpful pregnancy loss and stillbirth organizations. This is not a comprehensive list, but a selection of national and international resources that some of our contributors have found useful over the years.

Legislation, Health, and Public Policy

Adam's Song
Advocates for expanding fetal burial rights and provides child and pregnancy loss support: http://www.adamssong.net.

First Candle/SIDS Alliance
National network of health care providers, parents, caregivers, and researchers working on infant mortality and stillbirth. Supports national stillbirth legislation, and provides online resources, links to research, and twenty-four-hour hotline: (800) 221-7437, http://www.firstcandle.org.

Healthy Birth Day
Dedicated to the prevention of stillbirth and infant death through education, advocacy, and support. Created the Iowa Stillbirth Surveillance Project, the

first stillbirth registry, and is working to create a national stillbirth registry: http://www.healthybirthday.org.

Missing Angels Bill
Nationwide campaign to pass the Missing Angels Bill, a state-by-state push to issue modified birth certificates for stillbirths: http://www.missingangelsbill.org.

National Stillbirth Society
Parent-based group focused on raising awareness and preventing stillbirths through advocacy, education, and activism: http://www.stillnomore.org.

Prevention/Research/Education

BabyKick
Information on kick counting and the KickTrak, a digital kick-counting device: http://www.babykickalliance.org.

Count the Kicks
Informational posters, brochures, and kick-track cards for expectant parents and maternal health care providers. Developed public service announcement and awareness campaign for kick-counting and fetal movement awareness: http://www.countthekicks.org.

Group B Strep Association
Offers support and information, education, and awareness, and promotes testing and treatment of GBS: http://www.groupbstrep.org.

Group B Strep International
Focus includes all stages of development in which babies are susceptible to GBS infection, ranging from unborn babies in the first trimester to infants up to six months of age; information in English and Spanish: http://www.groupbstrepinternational.org.

International Society for the Study and Prevention of Perinatal and Infant Death (ISPID)
Group focused on advancing research and increasing knowledge about perinatal and infant health and mortality; hosts conferences and scientific workshops: http://www.ispid.org.

International Stillbirth Alliance (ISA)
Nonprofit coalition of organizations dedicated to understanding the causes and prevention of stillbirth. Its mission is to raise awareness, educate on recommended precautionary practices, and facilitate research on the prevention of stillbirth. ISA serves as a centralized resource for sharing information and connecting organizations and individuals; hosts biannual conference: http://www.stillbirthalliance.org.

Sidelines National Support Network
A network of support groups and support parents around the United States for women with complicated and high-risk pregnancies: http://www.sidelines.org.

Star Legacy Foundation
Offers education, birth planning support for families immediately after their loss, and fundraising for research, especially for cord- and placenta-related issues: http://www.starlegacyfoundation.org.

Trisomy 18 Foundation
Offers decision-making help, support, research, awareness, and education: http://www.trisomy18.org.

Twin-to-Twin Transfusion Syndrome Foundation (TTTS)
Resources for those diagnosed with TTTS during pregnancy or for those who have experienced loss of one or all babies due to TTTS; information in English, Spanish, French, and Dutch: 800-815-9211, http://www.tttsfoundation.org.

Bereavement and Support Networks

1st Breath
Offers compassion kits for hospitals and support to bereaved; advocates for increased monitoring, legislation, and awareness: http://www.1stbreath.org.

AMEND (Aiding Mothers and Fathers Experiencing Neonatal Death)
Offers free counseling services to parents who have lost an infant through miscarriage, stillbirth, or neonatal death: http://www.amendgroup.com.

Angel Names Association (ANA)
Dedicated to assisting families of stillborn children through programs designed to provide financial assistance for end-of-life expenses and counseling services, and funding for stillbirth research: http://www.angelnames.org.

Babycenter Forum
Online community forum/message board for those who need miscarriage, stillbirth, and infant-loss support: http://community.babycenter.com.

CLIMB (Center for Loss in Multiple Birth)
International group dedicated to providing parent-to-parent support for the death of one or more twins or multiples at any time from conception through early childhood. Also assists extended families, caregivers, and organizations: http://www.climb-support.org.

Compassionate Friends
National and local groups for families who have lost a child of any age: (877) 969-0010, http://www.compassionatefriends.org.

Feelings of the Fathers
Dedicated to fathers who are suffering the loss of their child; includes links and resources: http://www.thelaboroflove.com/forum/loss/fathers.html.

HAND (Helping After Neonatal Death)
Detailed online resources, support, and newsletter; regional support group meetings: http://www.handonline.org.

A Heartbreaking Choice
Resources, stories, and support for those who have terminated pregnancies due to genetic abnormalities: http://www.aheartbreakingchoice.com.

Hygeia Foundation
Institute for perinatal loss and bereavement: http://www.hygeia.org.

Journey of Hearts
An online healing site that combines elements of medicine, psychiatry, poetry, prose, and images to provide resources and support to those who have experienced loss: http://www.journeyofhearts.org.

MEND (Mommies Enduring Neonatal Death)
Support for those who have had a miscarriage, stillbirth, or early infant death; support group and newsletter: http://www.mend.org.

MISS Foundation
Dedicated to providing crisis and long-term support for parents who have lost a child; provides local support groups and online networking; active

in legislative and advocacy issues, community engagement, education, and research; hosts workshops and conferences: (623) 979-1000, http://www.missfoundation.org.

The Missing Angel Foundation
Stillbirth education and awareness, bulletin board community, online poetry, photo gallery, and chat room: http://www.missingangel.org.

Missing GRACE Foundation
Provides resources, support, and GRACE Care Baskets for families who have experienced pregnancy loss, infant loss, infertility, or adoption, and advocates for comprehensive, patient-focused prenatal care: (763) 497-0709, http://www.missinggrace.org.

Our Forever Babies
Offers a forum and chat room for anyone suffering pregnancy and infant loss: http://www.ourforeverbabies.com.

Perinatal Hospice
Organization that helps prepare families who face a fatal diagnosis during pregnancy by helping prepare a birth plan with parent wishes and/or a plan for baby's life, care, and death: http://www.perinatalhospice.org.

PLIDA (Pregnancy Loss and Infant Death Alliance)
A nationwide collective community of parents and health care professionals; annual conference: http://www.plida.org.

Pregnancy after Miscarriage (PAM)
Chat rooms, forums, and mailing lists for those who are pregnant, trying to get pregnant, or have had a baby after a loss: http://www.pamsupport.net.

Remembering Our Babies
The official site of Pregnancy and Infant Loss Remembrance Month (October) and Day (October 15); list of annual events and activities: http://www.pregnancyandinfantloss.org or http://www.october15th.com.

SHARE (A Source of Help in Airing and Resolving Experiences)
Pregnancy and infant loss support through newsletter, listserv, online support, and local support after a loss, including monthly meetings for subsequent pregnancies: (800) 821-6819, http://www.nationalshare.org.

SPALS (Subsequent Pregnancy after a Loss Support)
An online member support and resource group for subsequent pregnancies after the loss of a child due to miscarriage, selective termination, stillbirth, neonatal death, sudden infant death, or accidental death: http://www.spals.com.

Grieving and Remembering Resources

Angel Layettes
Donates blankets and baby outfits to hospitals. Seeks those who wish to sew or otherwise give to bereaved parents: http://www.angellayettes.org.

Babies Remembered
Newsletter/magazine, books, and support resources for parents and caregivers designed with the goal of helping improve the care families receive during and after the death of their child or loved one of any age; poetry, national/international updates, peer support parent training, consulting services for care providers and their facilities: (952) 476-1303, http://www.babiesremembered.org, http://www.helpwhenababydies.com, and http://www.wintergreenpress.com.

The Centering Corporation
Family-owned and -operated company dedicated to providing grief resources, books, and materials to those healing from loss: (402) 553-1200, http://www.centering.org.

Grief Watch
Bereavement resources, memorial products, and links for grieving families and professional caregivers: (503) 284-7426, http://www.griefwatch.com.

Mary Madeline Project
Donates infant/baby burial gowns and blankets made from donated wedding dresses to local hospitals for bereaved parents: http://www.marymadelineproject.org.

My Forever Child
Personalized remembrance jewelry and memorial keepsakes, specializing in miscarriage, stillbirth, and infant loss; custom handprint-footprint and photo jewelry from your child's actual images; newsletter and links to other resources: (888) 325-2828, http://www.myforeverchild.com.

Now I Lay Me Down to Sleep (NILMDTS)

Nonprofit organization of professional photographers offering the gift of a remembrance portrait for parents suffering the loss of a baby: http://www.nowilaymedowntosleep.org.

A Place to Remember

Support materials, resources, and links for those who have been touched by a crisis in pregnancy or the death of a baby: http://www.aplacetoremember.com.

Threads of Love

Gives blankets and baby clothing to hospitals for premature and ill infants as well as those who die before birth: http://www.threadsoflove.org.

Bereavement Training

Babies Remembered Consulting

Sherokee Ilse & Associates offers training and personalized consulting for care providers and their facilities; peer support parent training, companioning, birth planners, and parent advocates: http://www.babiesremembered.org.

Bereavement Services

Offers RTS (Resolve Through Sharing) training program for care providers: http://www.bereavementservices.org.

Center for Loss and Life Transition

Alan Wolfelt offers workshops and training seminars for caregivers and laypeople using a model of “companioning” versus “treating” people who are grieving: http://www.centerforloss.com.

International Resources

Bonnie Babes Foundation (Australia)

Provides twenty-four-hour telephone support and ongoing help for bereaved families; raises money for research: http://www.bbf.org.au.

Perinatal Bereavement Services (Canada)

Support services for families who have had a loss, as well as resources and seminars for health care providers: http://www.pbso.ca.

SANDS (UK/Australia/New Zealand)
Promotes awareness and understanding following the death of a baby from conception through infancy; newsletters, links to regional support groups, support, training, and resources; UK: http://www.uk-sands.org; Australia: http://www.sands.org.au; New Zealand: http://www.sands.org.nz.

SIDS and Kids (Australia)
Organization that researches causes of death, provides support for bereaved families, and offers community education to reduce incidence of SIDS and stillbirth. Offers bereavement support and counseling for families who have experienced stillbirth or the sudden and unexpected death of a child, whatever the cause, from twenty weeks' gestation to six years of age: http://www.sidsandkids.org.

Stillbirth Foundation (Australia)
Funds research and increases public awareness about stillbirth: http://www.stillbirthfoundation.org.au.

Events and Conferences

International Society for the Study and Prevention of Perinatal and Infant Death
http://www.ispid.org.

International Stillbirth Alliance Conference
http://www.stillbirthalliance.org.

MISS Foundation Conference
http://www.missfoundation.org/conference.

Pregnancy and Infant Loss Remembrance Day
October is Pregnancy and Infant Loss Awareness Month. October 15 is a national day of remembering, with candle lighting and memorial walks around the United States prior to and on October 15: http://www.october15th.com.

Pregnancy Loss and Infant Death Alliance (PLIDA)
http://www.perinatalbereavementconference.org.

Worldwide Candle Lighting
An opportunity to light a candle for a child of any age who has died; second Sunday in December: (877) 969-0010, http://www.compassionatefriends.org.

Books and Periodicals

Lorraine Ash, *Life Touches Life: A Mother's Story of Stillbirth and Healing*

Nina Bennett, *Forgotten Tears: A Grandmother's Journey through Grief*

Joanne Cacciatore, *Dear Cheyenne: A Journey into Grief*. Offers a pregnancy journal, self-help skills, poetry, and more.

Deborah L. Davis, PhD, *Empty Cradle, Broken Heart*

Maribeth Doerr, *For Better or Worse*

Ann Douglas and John R. Sussman, MD, *Trying Again: A Guide to Pregnancy after Miscarriage, Stillbirth, and Infant Loss*

Molly Fumia, *A Piece of My Heart: Living through the Grief of Miscarriage, Stillbirth, or Infant Death*

David Hansen, *I Hate This—A Play without the Baby*

Sherokee Ilse, *Empty Arms: Coping with Miscarriage, Stillbirth, and Infant Death*. Helps parents make critical decisions immediately following pregnancy and infant loss; includes a long list of resources. Updated and revised in 2008. Available in both English and Spanish.

Sherokee Ilse and Tim Nelson, *Couple Communication after a Baby Dies*

Amy Kuebelbeck, *Waiting with Gabriel: A Story of Cherishing a Baby's Brief Life*. A memoir about continuing a pregnancy with a terminal prenatal diagnosis.

Elizabeth McCracken, *An Exact Replica of a Figment of My Imagination*

Michelle Myers-Walters, *I Didn't Miscarry Her . . . She Died*

Tim Nelson, *A Guide for Fathers*

Corry Roach, *By Grace of Mourning*. Story of an infant that survived briefly.

Pat Schwiebert and Paul Kirk, *When Hello Means Goodbye: A Guide for Parents Whose Child Dies before Birth, at Birth, or Shortly after Birth*. Available in both English and Spanish.

Pat Schwiebert and Chuck DeKlyen, illustrated by Taylor Bills, *Tear Soup: A Recipe for Healing after Loss*. Available in both English and Spanish.

Laura Seftel, *Grief Unseen: Healing Pregnancy Loss through the Arts*

Books for Children

Elissa Al-Chokhachy, illustrated by Ulrike Graf, *An Angel with the Golden Glow*

Cathy Blanford, illustrated by Phyllis Childers, *Something Happened: A Book for Children and Parents Who Have Experienced Pregnancy Loss*

Linda Deymaz, *Mommy, Please Don't Cry: There Are No Tears in Heaven*

Rabbi Earl Grollman, *Talking about Death: A Dialogue between Parent and Child*

Marilyn Gryte, illustrated by Kristi McClendon, *No New Baby*; available at Centering Corporation; also in Spanish.

Patti Keough, *Remembering Our Baby*. A workbook for brothers and sisters whose baby dies before birth; available at Centering Corporation.

My Always Sister. A coloring book for children whose sibling dies before or shortly after birth; available at A Place to Remember.

Dan Schaefer, Christine Lyons, and David Peretz, MD, *How Do We Tell the Children? A Step-by-Step Guide for Helping Children Cope When a Loved One Dies*
Pat Schwiebert, illustrated by Taylor Bills, *Someone Came before You*
Pat Schwiebert, illustrated by Taylor Bills, *We Were Gonna Have a Baby, but We Had an Angel Instead*

Blogs

Babyloss Blog Directory
http://babylossdirectory.blogspot.com

Bereavement Magazine
http://www.bereavementmag.com

Broken Hearts, Living Hope newsletter
http://brokenheartslivinghope.homestead.com

Certificate of Birth Resulting in Stillbirth
http://cbrsbill.blogspot.com

Dead Baby Club
http://deadbabyclub.blogspot.com

Dr. Joanne Cacciatore
http://drjoanne.blogspot.com

Fathers Grieving Infant Loss
http://fathersgrievinginfantloss.blogspot.com

Glow in the Woods
http://www.glowinthewoods.com

Kara L. C. Jones
http://motherhenna.blogspot.com

Knocked Up, Knocked Down
http://knockedupknockeddown.blogspot.com

Love Reign over Me
http://scarletriver26.blogspot.com

Still Life 365
http://stilllife365.blogspot.com

Stirrup Queens
http://www.stirrup-queens.com

Notes

Chapter 3

1. You can read "My First Son, a True Memory" on the *New York Times* website at http://www.nytimes.com/2008/09/21/fashion/21love.html?_r=1.

Chapter 9

1. "The Phoenix Again." Copyright © 1988 by May Sarton, from *Collected Poems 1930–1993* by May Sarton. Used by permission of W. W. Norton & Company, Inc.

Chapter 10

1. Nancy Scheper-Hughes, *Death without Weeping: The Violence of Everyday Life in Brazil* (Berkeley: University of California Press, 1992).

Chapter 11

1. This is a common myth. Babies should not slow down, though the type of movement may change some. If the baby's pattern of movement and activeness changes (either becoming very, very active or slowing down), it is important to go to the hospital or clinic and be monitored over a period of time. For more about decreased fetal movement, see chapters 24 and 25.

2. Sherokee Ilse, *Empty Arms: Coping after Miscarriage, Stillbirth, and Infant Death*, 20th ed. (Maple Plain, MN: Wintergreen Press, 2008). Available through http://www.babiesremembered.org.

3. Alongside Ilse's group worked Sister Jane Marie Lamb and her SHARE parents, and soon after the Resolve through Sharing group from Wisconsin joined in, as well as professionals and parents from all over the United States. Ilse continues her work through consulting, at http://www.babiesremembered.org.

Chapter 20

1. The Secret Club Project (http://www.secretclubproject.org) was started by Laura Seftel, who also wrote the book *Grief Unseen: Healing Pregnancy Loss through the Arts* (Philadelphia: Jessica Kingsley Publishers, 2006).

2. This dictionary started as Jones's personal reaction to reading Sukie Miller and Doris Ober's book, *Finding Hope When a Child Dies: What Other Cultures Can Teach Us* (New York: Fireside, 2002). Upon reading the book, Jones discovered that the English language is ill-equipped to handle the death of a child. If your parents die, you are an orphan. If your partner dies, you are a widow or widower. But if your child dies, what are you? No words. So Jones set out to make her own language. After creating the first installment of this dictionary, Jones posted it, and many parents responded immediately and intimately with their own contributions. The ever-growing dictionary is housed at KotaPress. To contribute or read entries in the dictionary, visit http://www.kotapress.com/section_home/dictionary_intro.htm.

3. The free e-zines are available online in PDF format at http://www.kotapress.com/section_home/parentingZine_intro.htm.

4. Find out more about the Kindness Project in chapter 22 or at http://www.missfoundation.org/kindness/index.html.

5. Kiarash Khosrotehrani, Kirby L. Johnson, Dong Hyun Cha, Robert N. Salomon, and Diana W. Bianchi, "Transfer of Fetal Cells with Multilineage Potential to Maternal Tissue," *Journal of the American Medical Association* 292, no. 1 (2004): 75–80.

Chapter 21

1. You can read Pullen's "Calling All Angels" and "Hope with a Heartbeat" at the *San Francisco Chronicle* website at http://www.sfgate.com/pregnancyafterloss.

Chapter 24

1. J. A. Martin et al., "Births: Final Data for 2002," *National Vital Statistics Reports* 52, no. 10 (December 2003): 1–114; M. F. MacDorman and S. Kirmeyer, "The Challenge of Fetal Mortality," *NCHS Data Brief* 16 (2009).

2. M. Willinger, Chia-Wen Ko, and U. M. Reddy, "Racial Disparities in Stillbirth across Gestation in the United States," *American Journal of Obstetric Gynecology* 201 (2009): 469.e1–8.

3. M. Heron, "Leading Causes for 2004," *National Vital Statistics Reports* 56, no. 5 (November 2007).

4. G. C. S. Smith and Ruth Fretts, "Stillbirth," *The Lancet* 370 (2007): 1715–25.

5. Martin et al., "Births: Final Data for 2002"; MacDorman and Kirmeyer, "Challenge of Fetal Mortality."

6. Ruth Fretts, "Etiology and Prevention of Stillbirth," *American Journal of Obstetric Gynecology* 196 (2005): 1923–35.

7. MacDorman and Kirmeyer, "Challenge of Fetal Mortality."

8. MacDorman and Kirmeyer, "Challenge of Fetal Mortality."

9. Fretts, "Etiology and Prevention of Stillbirth"; Ruth Fretts, M. Boyd, R. H. Usher, and H. A. Usher, "The Changing Pattern of Fetal Death 1961–1988," *Obstetrics and Gynecology* 79 (1992): 35–39.

10. Y. Huang et al., "Determinants of Unexplained Antepartum Fetal Deaths," *Obstetrics and Gynecology* 95 (2000): 215–21.

11. U. M. Reddy, C. W. Ko, and M. Willinger, "Maternal Age and Risk of Stillbirth throughout Pregnancy in the United States," *American Journal of Obstetrics and Gynecology* 195 (2006): 764–70.

12. Customized growth charts are available free at http://www.gestation.net.

13. Reddy, Ko, and Willinger, "Maternal Age and Risk of Stillbirth."

14. R. N. Baergen, "Cord Abnormalities, Structural Lesions, Cord Accidents," *Seminars in Diagnostic Pathology* 24 (2007): 23–32.

15. Y. Oyelese and C. Ananth, "Placental Abruption," *Obstetrics and Gynecology* 108 (2006): 1005–15.

16. Smith and Fretts, "Stillbirth."

17. J. Robinson, B. Healy, T. Beatty, and A. Cohen, "The Optimal Gestational Age for Twin Delivery," *American Journal of Obstetrics and Gynecology* 193, no. 6 (2005): S183.

18. F. J. Korteweg et al., "Cytogenetic Analysis after Evaluation of 750 Fetal Deaths," *Obstetrics and Gynecology* 111 (2008): 865–74.

19. M. M. Lahra, A. Gordon, and H. E. Jeffery, "Chorioamnionitis and Fetal Response in Stillbirth," *American Journal of Obstetrics and Gynecology* 196 (2007): 229.e1–e4.

20. R. Romero and T. Chaiworapongsa, "Preterm Labor, Intrauterine Infection, and the Fetal Inflammatory Response Syndrome," *NeoReviews* 3, no. 5 (2002): e73.

21. See B. P. Zhu, R. T. Rolfs, B. E. Nangle, and J. M. Horan, "Effect of the Interval between Pregnancies on Perinatal Outcomes," *New England Journal of Medicine* 340 (1999): 589–94; G. C. S. Smith, J. P. Pell, and R. Dobbie, "Interpregnancy Interval and Risk of Preterm Birth and Neonatal Death: Retrospective Cohort Study," *British Medical Journal* 327 (2003): 313–16.

22. "Management of Stillbirth," *American Congress of Obstetricians and Gynecologists (ACOG) Practice Bulletin*, no. 102 (March 2009).

23. U. M. Reddy, "Prediction and Prevention of Recurrent Stillbirth," *Obstetrics and Gynecology* 110, no. 5 (2007): 1151–64.

24. Reddy, "Prediction and Prevention of Recurrent Stillbirth."

25. J. W. Weeks et al., "Antepartum Surveillance for a History of Stillbirth: When to Begin?" *American Journal of Obstetrics and Gynecology* 175 (1995): 486–92.

26. M. F. MacDorman and S. Kirmeyer, "The Challenge of Fetal Mortality," *NCHS Data Brief* 16 (2009).

27. J. F. Froen, "A Kick from Within—Fetal Movement Counting and the Cancelled Progress in Antenatal Care," *Journal of Perinatal Medicine* 32 (2004): 13.

28. A. Grant et al., "Routine Formal Fetal Movement Counting and Risk of Antepartum Late Death in Normally Formed Singletons," *Lancet* 2 (1989): 345.

29. A. E. Heazell and J. F. Froen, "Methods of Fetal Movement Counting and the Detection of Fetal Compromise," *Journal of Obstetrics and Gynaecology* 28, no. 2 (2008): 147–54.

30. O. O'Sullivan et al., "Predicting Poor Perinatal Outcome in Women Who Present with Decreased Fetal Movements," *Journal of Obstetrics and Gynaecology* 29, no. 8 (2009): 705–10.

31. J. V. Holm Tveit et al., "Reduction of Late Stillbirth with the Introduction of Fetal Movement Information and Guidelines: A Clinical Quality Improvement," *BMC Pregnancy and Childbirth* 32 (2009), http://www.biomedcentral.com/1471-2393/9/32.

32. E. Saastad et al., "Implementation of Uniform Information on Fetal Movement in a Norwegian Population Reduced Delayed Reporting of Decreased Fetal Movement in Primiparous Women—a Clinical Quality Improvement," *BMC Research Notes* 3 (2010): 2, http://www.biomedcentral.com/1756-0500/3/2.

Chapter 25

1. J. H. Collins, C. L. Collins, and C. C. Collins, "Umbilical Cord Accidents 2010," Pregnancy Institute, http://www.preginst.com/UCA_2010.pdf.

2. J. H. Collins, C. L. Collins, and C. C. Collins, "Umbilical Cord Accidents 2010."

3. M. M. Parast, C. P. Crum, and T. K. Boyd, "Placental Histologic Criteria for Umbilical Blood Flow Restriction in Unexplained Stillbirth," *Human Pathology* 39, no. 6 (2008): 948–53; P. Tantbirojn et al., "Gross Abnormalities of the Umbilical Cord: Related Placental Histology and Clinical Significance," *Placenta* 20, no. 12 (2009): 1083–88.

4. J. H. Collins and C. L. Collins, "The Human Umbilical Cord," in *The Placenta: Basic Science and Clinical Practice*, ed. J. Kingdom, E. Jauniaux, and S. O'Brien (London: RCOG Press, 2000), 319–29.

5. J. H. Collins, "Fetal Hiccups and the Umbilical Ring," *American Journal of Obstetric Gynecology* 165 (1991): 1161.

6. B. Wilson, "Sonography of the Placenta and Umbilical Cord," *Radiologic Technology* 79, no. 4 (2008): 333S–345S.

7. J. H. Collins, C. L. Collins, and C. C. Collins, "Umbilical Cord Accidents 2010."

8. E. Sadovsky and W. Z. Polishuk, "Fetal Movements in Utero: Nature, Assessment, Prognostic Value, Timing of Delivery," *Obstetrics and Gynecology* 50, no. 1 (1977): 49–55.

9. C. V. Towers, C. E. Juratsch, and T. J. Garite, "The Fetal Heart Monitor Tracing in Pregnancies Complicated by a Spontaneous Umbilical Cord Hematoma," *Journal of Perinatology* 29, no. 7 (2009): 517–20; A. Bord, S. Yagel, and D. V. Valsky, "Overburdened and Undernourished," *American Journal of Obstetric Gynecology* 197, no. 3 (2007): 324.e1–2.

10. B. Wilson, "Sonography of the Placenta and Umbilical Cord."

11. J. H. Collins, C. L. Collins, and C. C. Collins, "Umbilical Cord Accidents 2010."

12. One of the first published articles on UCA recurrence came out in 1956. The author, Dr. Vermelin, suggests that UCA can repeat in the same mom ("Multiple serres avec mort foetale à repetition," *Société d'Obstétrique et de Gynécologie de Nancy* [April 1956]: 192–94).

13. U. M. Reddy, "Prediction and Prevention of Recurrent Stillbirth," *Obstetrics and Gynecology* 110, no. 5 (2007): 1151–64.

14. J. H. Collins, "Pregnancy after Stillbirth and Home Fetal Heart Rate Monitoring via the Internet," Pregnancy Institute, http://www.preginst.com/case_study/case_study_6.html.

15. B. W. Bakotic et al., "Recurrent Umbilical Cord Torsion Leading to Fetal Death in 3 Subsequent Pregnancies," *Archives of Pathology and Laboratory Medicine* 124 (2000): 1352–55.

16. E. A. Friedman and R. K. Neff, "Hypertension-Hypotension in Pregnancy: Correlation with Fetal Outcome," *Journal of the American Medical Association* 239 (1978): 2249–51.

17. J. Warland, H. McCutcheon, and P. Baghurst, "Maternal Blood Pressure in Pregnancy and Third Trimester Stillbirth: A Case-Control Study," *American Journal of Perinatology* 25, no. 5 (2008): 311–17.

18. E. Hodgson and E. Norwitz, "Does Low Blood Pressure Increase the Risk of Stillbirth?" *Contemporary OB/GYN* (2006), http://www.contemporaryobgyn.net.

19. E. Bujold et al., "Reproducibility of First Trimester Three-Dimensional Placental Measurements in the Evaluation of Early Placental Insufficiency," *Journal of Obstetrics and Gynaecology Canada* 13, no. 12 (2009): 1144–48.

20. J. Warland, H. McCutcheon, and P. Baghurst, "Placental Position and Late Stillbirth: A Case-Control Study," *Journal of Clinical Nursing* 18 (2009): 1602–1606.

21. L. E. Kalanithi et al., "Intrauterine Growth Restriction and Placental Location," *Journal of Ultrasound in Medicine* 26 (2007): 1481–89.

22. K. V. Andersen et al., "Placenta Flow Index in Posterior Wall Placentas Measured With 99mtechnetium-Labelled Human Serum Albumin," *Clinical Physiology* 3, no. 6 (1983): 577–80.

23. S. Degani et al., "Myometrial Thickness in Pregnancy: Longitudinal Sonographic Study," *Journal of Ultrasound in Medicine* 17, no. 10 (1998): 661–65.

24. J. H. Collins et al., "Nuchal Cord: A Definition and a Study Associating Placental Location and Nuchal Cord Incidence," *Journal of the Louisiana State Medical Society* 143, no. 7 (1991): 18–23.

25. J. Gardosi, "Intrauterine Growth Restriction: New Standards for Assessing Adverse Outcome," *Best Practice & Research: Clinical Obstetrics & Gynaecology* 23 (2009): 741–49.

26. Gardosi, "Intrauterine Growth Restriction."

27. Gardosi, "Intrauterine Growth Restriction."

28. J. Gardosi, S. M. Kady, P. McGeown, A. Francis, and A. Tonks, "Classification of Stillbirth by Relevant Condition at Death (ReCoDe): Population Based Cohort Study," *British Medical Journal* 331 (2005): 1113–17.

29. Royal College of Obstetricians and Gynaecologists, "The Investigation and Management of the Small-for-Gestational-Age Fetus," *RCOG Green Top Guideline* No. 31, 2002, http://www.rcog.org.uk/womens-health/clinical-guidance/investigation-and-management-small-gestational-age-fetus-green-top-3.

30. Gardosi, "Intrauterine Growth Restriction."

31. J. Gardosi and A. Francis, "Controlled Trial of Fundal Height Measurement Plotted on Customised Antenatal Growth Charts," *British Journal of Obstetrics and Gynaecology* 106 (1999): 309–17.

32. Royal College of Obstetricians & Gynaecologists, "Investigation and Management."

33. Royal College of Obstetricians & Gynaecologists, "Investigation and Management."

34. Group B Strep International's website is http://www.groupbstrepinternational.org.

35. http://www.groupbstrepinternational.org.

36. F. T. Kraus, R. W. Redline, D. J. Gersell, D. M. Nelson, and J. M. Dicke, *Atlas of Nontumor Pathology: Placental Pathology*, 1st ed. (Washington, DC: American Registry of Pathology, Armed Forces Institute of Pathology, 2004).

37. Kraus et al., *Atlas of Nontumor Pathology*.

38. M. M. Parast, C. P. Crum, and T. K. Boyd, "Placental Histologic Criteria for Umbilical Blood Flow Restriction in Unexplained Stillbirth," *Human Pathology* 39, no. 6 (2008): 948–53.

39. D. R. Genest, "Estimating the Time of Death in Stillborn Fetuses: II. Histologic Evaluation of the Placenta: A Study of 71 Stillborns," *Obstetrics and Gynecology* 80, no. 4 (1992): 585–92.

40. To find out more or to see how you can help expand the stillbirth registry in your area, contact Healthy Birthday at info@healthybirthday.org.

41. Abstracts 5 and 27, *American Journal of Obstetrics and Gynecology* 201, no. 6 (2009); Abstract 339, *Reproductive Sciences* 17, no. 3 supplement (2010).

Bibliography

Andersen, K. V., O. Munck, J. F. Larsen, and H. Kjeldsen. "Placenta Flow Index in Posterior Wall Placentas Measured with 99mtechnetium-Labelled Human Serum Albumin." *Clinical Physiology* 3, no. 6 (1983): 577–80.

Baergen, R. N. "Cord Abnormalities, Structural Lesions, Cord Accidents." *Seminars in Diagnostic Pathology* 24 (2007): 23–32.

Bakotic, B. W., T. Boyd, R. Poppiti, and S. Pflueger. "Recurrent Umbilical Cord Torsion Leading to Fetal Death in 3 Subsequent Pregnancies." *Archives of Pathology and Laboratory Medicine* 124 (2000): 1352–55.

Bord, A., S. Yagel, and D. V. Valsky. "Overburdened and Undernourished." *American Journal of Obstetric Gynecology* 197, no. 3 (2007): 324.e1–2.

Bujold, E., M. Effendi, M. Girard, K. Gouin, J. C. Forest, B. Couturier, and Y. Giguère. "Reproducibility of First Trimester Three-Dimensional Placental Measurements in the Evaluation of Early Placental Insufficiency." *Journal of Obstetrics and Gynaecology Canada* 13, no. 12 (2009): 1144–48.

Collins, J. H. "Fetal Hiccups and the Umbilical Ring." *American Journal of Obstetric Gynecology* 165 (1991): 1161.

———. "Pregnancy after Stillbirth and Home Fetal Heart Rate Monitoring via the Internet." Pregnancy Institute, http://www.preginst.com/case_study/case_study_6.html.

Collins, J. H., and C. L. Collins. "The Human Umbilical Cord." In *The Placenta: Basic Science and Clinical Practice*, edited by J. Kingdom, E. Jauniaux, and S. O'Brien, 319–29. London: RCOG Press, 2000.

Collins, J. H., C. L. Collins, and C. C. Collins. "Umbilical Cord Accidents 2010." Pregnancy Institute, http://www.preginst.com/UCA_2010.pdf.

Collins, J. H., D. Geddes, C. L. Collins, and L. De Angelis. "Nuchal Cord: A Definition and a Study Associating Placental Location and Nuchal Cord Incidence." *Journal of the Louisiana State Medical Society* 143, no. 7 (1991): 18–23.

Degani, S., Z. Leibovitz, I. Shapiro, R. Gonen, and G. Ohel. "Myometrial Thickness in Pregnancy: Longitudinal Sonographic Study." *Journal of Ultrasound in Medicine* 17, no. 10 (1998): 661–65.

Fretts, Ruth. "Etiology and Prevention of Stillbirth." *American Journal of Obstetric Gynecology* 196 (2005): 1923–35.

Fretts, Ruth, M. Boyd, R. H. Usher, and H. A. Usher. "The Changing Pattern of Fetal Death 1961–1988." *Obstetrics and Gynecology* 79 (1992): 35–39.

Friedman, E. A., and R. K. Neff. "Hypertension-Hypotension in Pregnancy: Correlation with Fetal Outcome." *Journal of the American Medical Association* 239 (1978): 2249–51.

Froen, J. F. "A Kick from Within—Fetal Movement Counting and the Cancelled Progress in Antenatal Care." *Journal of Perinatal Medicine* 32 (2004): 13.

Gardosi, J. "Intrauterine Growth Restriction: New Standards for Assessing Adverse Outcome." *Best Practice & Research: Clinical Obstetrics & Gynaecology* 23 (2009): 741–49.

Gardosi, J., and A. Francis. "Controlled Trial of Fundal Height Measurement Plotted on Customised Antenatal Growth Charts." *British Journal of Obstetrics and Gynaecology* 106 (1999): 309–17.

Gardosi, J., S. M. Kady, P. McGeown, A. Francis, and A. Tonks. "Classification of Stillbirth by Relevant Condition at Death (ReCoDe): Population Based Cohort Study." *British Medical Journal* 331 (2005): 1113–17.

Genest, D. R. "Estimating the Time of Death in Stillborn Fetuses: II. Histologic Evaluation of the Placenta; A Study of 71 Stillborns." *Obstetrics and Gynecology* 80, no. 4 (1992): 585–92.

Grant, A., D. Elbourne, L. Valentin, and S. Alexander. "Routine Formal Fetal Movement Counting and Risk of Antepartum Late Death in Normally Formed Singletons." *Lancet* 2 (1989): 345.

Haws, Rachel, Mohammad Y. Yakoob, Tanya Soomro, Esme V. Menezes, Gary L. Darmstadt, and Zulfiqar A. Bhutta. "Reducing Stillbirths: Screening and Monitoring during Pregnancy and Labour." *BMC Pregnancy and Childbirth* 9, Supplement 1 (2009), http://www.biomedcentral.com/1471-2393/9/S1/S5.

Heazell, A. E., and J. F. Froen. "Methods of Fetal Movement Counting and the Detection of Fetal Compromise." *Journal of Obstetrics and Gynaecology* 28, no. 2 (2008): 147–54.

Heron, M. "Leading Causes for 2004." *National Vital Statistics Reports* 56, no. 5 (November 2007).

Hodgson, E., and E. Norwitz. "Does Low Blood Pressure Increase the Risk of Stillbirth?" *Contemporary OB/GYN* (2006), http://www.contemporaryobgyn.net.

Holm Tveit, J. V., E. Saastad, B. Stray-Pedersen, P. E. Bordahl, V. Flenady, R. Fretts, and J. F. Froen. "Reduction of Late Stillbirth with the Introduction of Fetal Movement Information and Guidelines: A Clinical Quality Improvement." *BMC Pregnancy and Childbirth* 32 (2009), http://www.biomedcentral.com/1471-2393/9/32.

Huang, D. Y., R. H. Usher, M. S. Kramer, H. Yang, L. Morin, and R. Fretts. "Determinants of Unexplained Antepartum Fetal Deaths." *Obstetrics and Gynecology* 95 (2000): 215–21.

Ilse, Sherokee. *Empty Arms: Coping after Miscarriage, Stillbirth, and Infant Death*. 20th ed. Maple Plain, MN: Wintergreen Press, 2008.

Kalanithi, L. E., J. L. Illuzzi, V. B. Nossov, Y. Frisbaek, S. Abdel-Razeq, J. A. Copel, and E. R. Norwitz. "Intrauterine Growth Restriction and Placental Location." *Journal of Ultrasound in Medicine* 26 (2007): 1481–89.

Khosrotehrani, Kiarash, Kirby L. Johnson, Dong Hyun Cha, Robert N. Salomon, and Diana W. Bianchi. "Transfer of Fetal Cells with Multilineage Potential to Maternal Tissue." *Journal of the American Medical Association* 292, no. 1 (2004): 75–80.

Korteweg, F. J., K. Bouman, J. J. Erwich, A. Timmer, N. J. Veeger, J. M. Ravise, T. H. Nigman, and J. P. Holm. "Cytogenetic Analysis after Evaluation of 750 Fetal Deaths." *Obstetrics and Gynecology* 111 (2008): 865–74.

Kraus, F. T., R. W. Redline, D. J. Gersell, D. M. Nelson, and J. M. Dicke. *Atlas of Nontumor Pathology: Placental Pathology*. 1st ed. (Washington, DC: American Registry of Pathology, Armed Forces Institute of Pathology, 2004).

Lahra, M. M., A. Gordon, and H. E. Jeffery. "Chorioamnionitis and Fetal Response in Stillbirth." *American Journal of Obstetrics and Gynecology* 196 (2007): 229.e1–e4.

Llurba, Elisa, Elena Carreras, Eduard Gratacos, Miquel Juan, Judith Astor, Angels Vives, Eduard Hermosilla, Ines Calero, Pilar Millan, Barbara Garcia-Valdecasas, and Lluis Cabero. "Maternal History and Uterine Artery Doppler in the Assessment of Risk for Development of Early- and Late-Onset Preeclampsia and Intrauterine Growth Restriction." *Obstetrics and Gynecology International* online (e-pub May 27, 2009), doi:10.1155/2009/275613.

MacDorman, M. F., and S. Kirmeyer. "The Challenge of Fetal Mortality." *NCHS Data Brief* 16 (2009).

Malchiodi, Cathy. *Art Therapy Sourcebook*. 2nd ed. New York: McGraw-Hill, 2006.

"Management of Stillbirth." *American Congress of Obstetricians and Gynecologists (ACOG) Practice Bulletin* no. 102 (March 2009).

Martin, Joyce A., Brady E. Hamilton, Paul D. Sutton, Stephanie J. Ventura, Fay Menacker, and Martha L. Munson. "Births: Final Data for 2002." *National Vital Statistics Reports* 52, no. 10 (December 2003): 1–114.

Miller, Sukie, and Doris Ober. *Finding Hope When a Child Dies: What Other Cultures Can Teach Us*. New York: Fireside, 2002.

Naidus, Beverly. *Arts for Change: Teaching outside the Frame*. Oakland, CA: New Village Press, 2009.

O'Sullivan, O., G. Stephen, E. Martindale, and A. E. Heazell. "Predicting Poor Perinatal Outcome in Women Who Present with Decreased Fetal Movements." *Journal of Obstetrics and Gynaecology* 29, no. 8 (2009): 705–10.

Oyelese, Y., and C. Ananth. "Placental Abruption." *Obstetrics and Gynecology* 108 (2006): 1005–15.

Parast, M. M., C. P. Crum, and T. K. Boyd. "Placental Histologic Criteria for Umbilical Blood Flow Restriction in Unexplained Stillbirth." *Human Pathology* 39, no. 6 (2008): 948–53.

Pullen, Suzanne. "Calling All Angels." *San Francisco Chronicle*, http://www.sfgate.com/pregnancyafterloss.

———. "Hope with a Heartbeat." *San Francisco Chronicle*, http://www.sfgate.com/pregnancyafterloss.

Reddy, U. M. "Prediction and Prevention of Recurrent Stillbirth." *Obstetrics and Gynecology* 110, no. 5 (2007): 1151–64.

Reddy, U. M., C. W. Ko, and M. Willinger. "Maternal Age and Risk of Stillbirth throughout Pregnancy in the United States." *American Journal of Obstetrics and Gynecology* 195 (2006): 764–70.

Robinson, J., B. Healy, T. Beatty, and A. Cohen. "The Optimal Gestational Age for Twin Delivery." *American Journal of Obstetrics and Gynecology* 193, no. 6 (2005): S183.

Romero, R., and T. Chaiworapongsa. "Preterm Labor, Intrauterine Infection, and the Fetal Inflammatory Response Syndrome." *NeoReviews* 3, no. 5 (2002): e73.

Royal College of Obstetricians and Gynaecologists. "The Investigation and Management of the Small-for-Gestational-Age Fetus." *RCOG Green Top Guideline* no. 31, 2002, http://www.rcog.org.uk/womens-health/clinical-guidance/investigation-and-management-small-gestational-age-fetus-green-top-3.

Saastad, E., J. V. Holm Tveit, V. Flenady, B. Stray-Pedersen, R. Fretts, P. E. Bordahl, and J. F. Froen. "Implementation of Uniform Information on Fetal Movement in a Norwegian Population Reduced Delayed Reporting of Decreased Fetal Movement in Primiparous Women—a Clinical Quality Improvement." *BMC Research Notes* 3 (2010): http://www.biomedcentral.com/1756-0500/3/2.

Sadovsky, E., and W. Z. Polishuk. "Fetal Movements in Utero: Nature, Assessment, Prognostic Value, Timing of Delivery." *Obstetrics and Gynecology* 50, no. 1 (1977): 49–55.

Scheper-Hughes, Nancy. *Death without Weeping: The Violence of Everyday Life in Brazil*. Berkeley: University of California Press, 1992.

Seftel, Laura. *Grief Unseen: Healing Pregnancy Loss through the Arts*. Philadelphia: Jessica Kingsley Publishers, 2006.

Smith, G. C. S., and Ruth Fretts. "Stillbirth." *The Lancet* 370 (2007): 1715–25.

Smith, G. C. S., J. P. Pell, and R. Dobbie. "Interpregnancy Interval and Risk of Preterm Birth and Neonatal Death: Retrospective Cohort Study." *British Medical Journal* 327 (2003): 313–16.

Stubblefield, Phillip, Dean V. Coonrod, Uma M. Reddy, Raja Sayegh, Wanda Nicholson, Daniel F. Rychlik, and Brian W. Jack. "The Clinical Content of Preconception Care: Reproductive History." *American Journal of Obstetrics and Gynecology* Supplement (December 2008): S373–83.

Tantbirojn, P., A. Saleemuddin, K. Sirois, C. P. Crum, T. K. Boyd, S. Tworoger, and M. M. Parast. "Gross Abnormalities of the Umbilical Cord: Related Placental Histology and Clinical Significance." *Placenta* 30, no. 12 (2009): 1083–88.

Towers, C. V., C. E. Juratsch, and T. J. Garite. "The Fetal Heart Monitor Tracing in Pregnancies Complicated by a Spontaneous Umbilical Cord Hematoma." *Journal of Perinatology* 29, no. 7 (2009): 517–20.

Vermelin, M. H. "Multiples serres avec mort foetale à repetition." *Societe d'Obstétrique et de Gynécologie de Nancy* (April 1956): 192–94.

Warland, J. "Is Maternal Hypotension during Pregnancy and/or Posterior Located Placenta Associated with Increased Risk of Stillbirth? A Case-Control Study." PhD diss., University of Adelaide, 2006.

Warland, J., H. McCutcheon, and P. Baghurst. "Maternal Blood Pressure in Pregnancy and Third Trimester Stillbirth: A Case-Control Study." *American Journal of Perinatology* 25, no. 5 (2008): 311–17.

———. "Placental Position and Late Stillbirth: A Case-Control Study." *Journal of Clinical Nursing* 18 (2009): 1602–1606.

Weeks, J. W., T. Asrat, M. A. Morgan, M. Nageotte, S. J. Thomas, and R. K. Freeman. "Antepartum Surveillance for a History of Stillbirth: When to Begin?" *American Journal of Obstetrics and Gynecology* 175 (1995): 486–92.

Willinger, M., Chia-Wen Ko, and U. M. Reddy. "Racial Disparities in Stillbirth across Gestation in the United States." *American Journal of Obstetric Gynecology* 201 (2009): 469.e1–8.

Wilson, B. "Sonography of the Placenta and Umbilical Cord." *Radiologic Technology* 79, no. 4 (2008): 333S–345S.

Zhu, B. P., R. T. Rolfs, B. E. Nangle, and J. M. Horan. "Effect of the Interval between Pregnancies on Perinatal Outcomes." *New England Journal of Medicine* 340 (1999): 589–94.

Index

Abbey, Amy, xx, 125–33, 179, 241
abortion, 18
adoption, xix, 42–44, 55
advice from others, 26, 105–6, 111; not to see the baby, 110. *See also* comments from others
Andersen, Hans Christian, 59
anencephaly, xx, 14, 18, 110
Angel Layettes, 178
angel, referring to stillborn baby as, 4, 23, 44, 65, 68, 95–100, 157, 164, 170
anger: as catalyst for change, 73, 132; caused by others, 76, 89, 92, 112; at God, 122; at health care provider, 8; at medical community, 10; at oneself, 17; as part of the grief process, 40, 49, 144; repression of, 75–76
anniversaries. *See* birthdays
antidepressant, 116
anxiety, 122, 126, 129, 155; fetal surveillance to ease, 192; not increased by education about fetal movement, 195. *See also* fear
art and grief. *See* visual arts and grief
Ash, Lorraine, 148
ashes/cremains, 27, 75, 160, 175; keeping the, 17, 45
asking "Why my baby?" 4, 21, 23, 92, 112
assisted reproductive technology, 66
autopsy, 8, 186, 201, 212–13

Baby Kick Alliance, 218
babyloss community, 49, 92–93, 125, 128, 130, 140, 146, 165–68
baby's body: holding/seeing, 14, 20, 31–32, 35, 51–52, 58, 68, 104, 156–57; regrets about not having enough time with, 26, 59, 72–73, 98. *See also* memories
baby showers, 72, 87–88, 129, 146, 163
Back to Sleep campaign, 11, 197
baptism/infant blessing, xviii, 39
Bennett, Nina, xix, 103–7, 241–42
birth certificate, 22, 24, 39, 142; death certificate instead of a, 22, 142. *See also* certificate of birth resulting in stillbirth
birthdays: including family and friends in, 79; others forgetting, 90;

preparing for, 74, 174–76; ways of remembering, 51, 55, 74–77, 95, 101, 122, 140
bleeding during pregnancy, 17, 188, 193–94, 205, 208
blood clotting problems, 191
blood pressure, maternal. *See* maternal blood pressure
burial, 22, 26, 37–38, 39, 68, 111–12, 175; cultural differences and, 68. *See also* funeral/memorial service

Cacciatore, Joanne, xix, 19–28, 148, 178–79, 225, 226, 242, 244
Caesarian section. *See* C-section
Caring Arms Support Group, 115
causes of stillbirth. *See* stillbirth, causes of
CDC (Centers for Disease Control), 214
certificate of birth resulting in stillbirth, 24, 218, 226
changes: in faith, 53; in listening to others' stories, 4, 49; in perspective, 5, 13, 44, 106–7, 120, 123–24, 140, 150; in priorities, 73–74, 112–13, 120, 145; in self, 22, 32, 34, 41, 73, 106–7, 117. *See also* couples, faith, friends, grief
children. *See* subsequent pregnancy, subsequent children, living children, and telling living children
chorioamonitis, 66
Christmas. *See* holidays
chromosomal abnormalities, 189–90, 192
Collins, Jason, 199, 201–3, 204
comments from others: helpful, 92–93, 111–12; hurtful, 2, 4, 18, 23, 40, 76, 89, 142; online, 18
confusion. *See* numbness and shock
control: over destiny, 119; recognizing lack of, 32, 106, 121, 123, 152; and grief, 74, 123, 176. *See also* fear
cord accident. *See* umbilical cord accident
Count the Kicks, 218
Couple Communication after a Baby Dies (Nelson and Ilse), xx, 245
couples: communication, 54, 73, 85, 110, 122; differences between males and females, 17, 40, 54, 76–77, 131; and sexual intimacy, 81; taking turns with grieving, 47
crazy: feeling, xiv, 45, 53, 73, 112, 114; others thinking you are, 27, 33; worries about feeling, 112
creativity, 141–49, 151, 175; tapping into your, 177–78, 181–82. *See also* visual arts and grief
C-section, 51, 54, 163, 197, 203–4, 208
cultural differences in bereavement, 65, 68

D & C (dilation and curettage), 14, 42, 128, 129
death of baby. *See* stillbirth
Dear Cheyenne (Cacciatore), 225
decreased fetal movement. See fetal movement, decrease in
denial, 20, 40, 58, 98, 105; in subsequent pregnancy, 54, 129. *See also* anger, repression of
depression, 32, 40, 72, 122, 124, 176
diabetes, 188, 192–93, 215; gestational, 191
divide life into before and after the loss, 2–5, 31, 119–20; not wanting to, 67
doctor. *See* health care provider
Down syndrome, 9, 11, 190
drug use, maternal, 188

emptiness, 3, 34, 54, 110, 160, 140; arms, 40, 73, 128, 135, 139, 179; belly, 22, 29, 46, 159. *See also Empty Arms*
Empty Arms (Ilse), xix, 73, 79, 225, 243
envy. *See* jealousy

faith, 22, 92, 96, 120; impacted by loss, xix, 52–53, 59, 112, 122
fathers, 66, 77; coping with feelings, 15–16, 35; and crying, 51, 59, 110; feelings of responsibility, 30; invisible grief, 76, 131; isolation, 91, 110; resources for, 220
Father's Day. *See* holidays, Mother's Day/Father's Day
Fathers Grieving Infant Loss (blog), 226
fear: awaiting word about baby, 20, 96; the baby will be forgotten, 4, 142–43, 173; of losing control of emotions, 123; of social settings, 47, 122; in subsequent pregnancy, 54, 61, 75, 129
fetal cells in mother's body after delivery, 146, 146n5, 161
fetal death. *See* stillbirth
fetal demise. *See* stillbirth
fetal distress, 51
fetal growth chart, customized, 188, 188n11, 210–11
fetal growth restriction. *See* intrauterine growth restriction (IUGR)
fetal hiccupping, 201
fetal movement: and cord accidents, 201–2; decrease in, 72, 72n1, 88–89, 96, 194, 201; medical response to decreased, 195–7; sleep patterns and, 195–96, 207; studies about, 194; in subsequent pregnancy, 192; when to call your doctor about, 196–97. *See also* kick counting
fetal to maternal hemorrhage, 213
financial concerns, 39, 219
First Candle/SIDS Alliance, 131, 178, 217, 241, 245
Flores, Marion, xix, 37–44, 242
forget: pressure from others to, 26, 112; that the baby is dead, 46, 48; unwilling to, 22, 60, 67, 98, 101, 155, 168, 173
Forgotten Tears (Bennett), xix, 225, 241
Francis, Saint, 22
frequency of stillbirth. *See* stillbirth, frequency of
Fretts, Ruth, xx, 10–11, 185–97
friends, 40, 46, 48, 107, 120, 142, 147; reactions of, 40; support from, 51, 91, 167; withdrawal from, 91
funeral home workers, 58–59, 107
funeral/memorial service, 37, 99–100, 107, 175; community, 74, 175; regrets about, 111

Gardosi, Jason, 200, 210–11
"getting over" your baby, 34, 35, 41, 145, 147, 180
Glow in the Woods (blog), xix, 226, 246
Goldenbach, Alan, xix, 7–12, 243
Graham, Rachel, xix, 51–55, 243
grandparents, 37–38, 103–7
grief: after stillbirth versus other types of loss, xv, xix, 13–14; and creativity, 141–49; duration of, 3, 149–50; health providers and, 115–16; intensity of, 49, 89, 139; no right or wrong way to move through, 150; patience with your, 147, 149–50, 174; physical symptoms of, 3, 183; and poverty, 65; process of, 31, 40, 100, 106, 107, 111, 139, 144–45; relieved by subsequent live birth, 17, 129; seeking validation of your, 105–6; talking with others about your, 176; trying to avoid the process of, 111; unanticipated, 100, 132, 174, 180; unpredictability of, 5. *See also* anger, denial, fear, guilt, jealousy, numbness and shock, visual arts and grief
group B strep (GBS), 190, 211–12
Group B Strep International, 218
A *Guide for Fathers* (Nelson), 225
guilt, 40, 50, 66–67, 110–11, 112, 139

Haggard, Cheryl, 148
Hasegawa, Junichi, 199, 203–4
health care providers, 2, 8, 39, 110–11, 115; anger toward, 8; conversations with, 144–45; reactions of, 29, 136, 157; resistance to changes in stillbirth procedure, 113–16; sharing research with, 207; support from, 14, 39, 52, 113
helplessness, 9, 106, 121, 123
high-risk pregnancy, 8, 188–89, 192, 219
Hlavsa, David, xix, 13–18, 243
holidays, 1, 76, 78, 95, 143, 145–46, 176; difficulty during, 41, 100–101; Mother's Day/Father's Day, 82, 84, 143
honoring your baby's memory, 74, 79, 100, 173–80
hospital staff. *See* health care providers
"How many children do you have?" 18, 45, 68
husband. *See* father and couples

Ilse, Sherokee, xiv, xx, 71–80, 176, 223, 225, 243
incompetent cervix, 38, 129
induced labor: in cases of decreased fetal movement, 196–97; in previable pregnancies, 127–28, 185; in stillbirth, 14, 58, 66, 97, 122, 137
infection: common identifiable cause of stillbirth, 186, 215; and fetal growth restriction, 188, 209; summary of, 190, 211–12; uterine, 66
infertility, 16, 41–42, 109, 220, 221
insensitive comments from others. *See* comments from others
insomnia. *See* sleep
intrauterine growth restriction (IUGR), 187–88, 196, 209–11; risk of recurrence, 192
Iowa Stillbirth Surveillance Project, 213–14, 217
isolation, 11, 30, 47, 61, 105, 122, 135, 139–40

jealousy, 92, 137, 138
jewelry, 50, 175, 178, 222. *See also* mementos
Jones, Kara L. C. , xx, 141n2, 141–50, 177, 181–83, 226, 243–44
journaling, xiii–xiv, 48, 130, 141–42, 151, 175, 177; exercises, 181–82
Journeys (Abbey), xx, 131, 241

keepsakes. *See* mementos
kick counting, 11, 187, 192, 194–96, 202
kindness cards, 143, 178–79
Knocked Up, Knocked Down (LeMoine), xix, 226, 244
KotaPress, 141, 144–45, 146
Krahling, Kelley, xix, 29–35, 244

labor: difficulty of being in a maternity ward, 14, 31, 137; with stillbirth, xvii, 14, 20, 30, 38, 51, 58, 66, 98, 110, 128, 156; with subsequent pregnancy, 62–63
lactation. *See* milk
legislation, 24–25
LeMoine, Monica Murphy, xix, 81–86, 244
Lewis, C. S. 26
living children, 17, 44, 67, 77, 177; bittersweetness and, 34, 46–47, 49–50; telling about the stillbirth, 50, 76–77, 101, 147. *See also* stillbirth, younger siblings; stillbirth, older siblings; and subsequent children
loneliness. *See* isolation
low birth weight babies. *See* intrauterine growth restriction (IUGR)

Malchiodi, Cathy, 143, 146, 149, 181–82

March of Dimes, 178
marriage. *See* couples
maternal age as risk factor in stillbirth rates. *See* stillbirth, risk factors
maternal blood pressure, 188, 192, 205–7, *206*
McCracken, Elizabeth, xiii–xv, 225
McVicar, Candy, xix, 87–93, 244
media representations of stillbirth, 32–33, 74
mementos, 39, 45, 174–75; not having, 72–73
memorial, 175–76
memorializing the baby, xx, 100–101, 107, 117, 142, 174–80
memorial service. *See* funeral/memorial service
memories: creating 78, 98, 104, 116; dwelling on, 57; fading over time, 29, 139–40; importance of, 33, 79, 92, 112, 174–76; not having, 34; of pregnancy, 84; revisiting, 69, 75; sharing with others, 176
midwives. *See* health care providers
milk, 22, 52, 67, 139
miscarriage, 72, 77, 88, 97, 120, 126, 137, 139, 148, 189; resources for those who have suffered a, 219–22, 225
MISS Foundation, xix, 23, 146, 178, 220–21, 242
MISS Foundation Conference, 146, 150, 224
Missing GRACE Foundation, 93, 221, 244
Mother's Day. *See* holidays
multiples, xix, 66–67, 120, 138–39, 189, 220

naïveté, 46, 71–72, 120, 137
name, 20, 23, 50, 59, 111, 128; being said and remembered, 3, 76, 142–43, 166, 173, 176; helping others in your baby's, 75, 143, 178
National Institute of Child Health and Human Development (NICHD), 204, 214
National Institutes of Health, 25
National Stillbirth Registry, 214
Nelson, Tim, xx, 119–24, 245
no known cause of stillbirth. *See* unknown cause of stillbirth
nonstress test (NST): and cord anomalies, 204, 202; definition of, 187, 194; reassurance from, 207, 209; use of, 129
Now I Lay Me Down to Sleep (NILMDTS), 148, 223
nuchal cord, 202–3, 209
numbness and shock, 51, 57, 60, 68, 89, 98, 104, 110, 122, 136
nursery, 19, 40, 72, 112
nurses. *See* health care providers

other children. *See* living children and subsequent children

Parast, Mana, 200, 212–13
parenting while grieving, 31, 46–50, 100, 177
Paris, Jenell Williams, xix, 65–69, 245
past generations and stillbirth. *See* stillbirth, historical responses to
photographs of the baby, 27, 34, 39, 52, 53, 104, 113–14, 160; causing discomfort to others, 11, 113, 147; inclusion in a memory box, 175; medical use of, 189; not having, 72, 98, 122. *See also* mementos; Now I Lay Me Down to Sleep (NILMDTS)
placenta: importance in autopsy, 190, 212–13; infection and, 190, 211–12; and intrauterine growth restriction, 209–10; and maternal blood pressure, 205–6; position of the, 208–9; previa, 208; problems with,

188, 207–9; structure of, 207–8; and umbilical cord accidents, 202, 203
placental abruption, 10, 17, 186–89, 197, 199, 208, 213
poetry, 60–61, 75, 175, 182; as expression of deep feelings, 76, 142–43, 151; inclusion in memory box, 175; prompt for writing, 182
post-date pregnancy, 109, 186, 196
powerlessness. *See* control over destiny
prayer, 38, 66, 75, 92, 96, 114; trying to understand the loss through, 53
preeclampsia, 8, 10, 188, 193, 208, 210, 212
Pregnancy and Infant Loss Remembrance Month (October), 73–74, 175
Pregnancy Institute, the, 199, 201, 204
pregnancy losses, other: definition vis-à-vis stillbirth, xviii, 139, 215; miscarriage, 17, 72, 77, 97, 120, 137; not included in stillbirth statistics, 185; society's responses to, 67
pregnant friends and family, 90, 92, 153–65; 215
preventing stillbirth, 187, 194, 202
Pullen, Suzanne, xx, 151–70, 175, 245

rates of stillbirth. *See* stillbirth, frequency of
reason for stillbirth. *See* stillbirth, causes of
regret, 11, 26, 72, 97, 98; about not seeing the baby, 110, 113
reincarnation, 59–63
relatives. *See* friends, grandparents, and stillbirth and extended family
religion. *See* faith
resentment. *See* anger and jealousy
resolution, 63, 67, 69; not aiming for, 67, 106; seeing positives, 41, 44, 50, 77
Resolve Through Sharing, 73n3, 114, 223
Rich, Adrienne, 19
risk of recurrence of stillbirth. See stillbirth, risk of recurrence. *See also* umbilical cord accidents, recurrence
rituals, 13, 19, 177

SANDS (Stillbirth and Neonatal Death Society), 52–55, 224, 243
Sarton, May, 60
Scheper-Hughes, Nancy, 65, 68
Seftel, Laura, 141, 148
SHARE (A Source of Help in Airing and Resolving Experiences), 73n3, 178, 221–22
sharing your story, 116, 126–32, 179–80. *See also* telling others and writing after stillbirth
shock. *See* numbness and shock
siblings. *See* stillbirth, older siblings; stillbirth, younger siblings; subsequent children; and living children
silence about stillbirth, 4, 7–9, 10, 23–24, 25, 40, 142, 144
SIDS (Sudden Infant Death Syndrome), 9, 11, 197
signs from the baby, 60, 107, 164
Skipper, Kathleen, xx, 109–17, 245–46
sleep, 16, 20; back to, 11; and maternal low blood pressure, 201, 206; nightmares during, 105; positions during pregnancy, 207
smoking, maternal, 188, 193, 197, 215
societal responses to stillbirth. *See* stillbirth, societal responses to
spirituality. *See* faith
stillbirth: and black women, 186; books, xviii, 7–8, 225–26; causes of, 10, 186–90, 215; definition of early vs. late stillbirth, 185; extended family responses to, 37, 40, 87–93, 97, 100, 120, 176; hearing other people's stories of, xiv–xv, 17–18,

50, 138–40; historical responses to, 144; impact on partner relationship, 40, 47, 54, 76, 81, 110–11, 131; lack of awareness about, 2, 3, 88, 137; and older siblings, 46–47, 58, 60, 100; frequency of stillbirth, 149, 185–86; risk factors for, 187, 193; risk of recurrence of, 192–93; societal responses to, 23, 67, 91–92, 105; standardized reporting of, 24, 212, 213–14; U.S. data on, xviii, 9, 185–86, 214; and younger siblings, 68, 76–77, 126. *See also* emptiness; fathers; grief; labor; silence about stillbirth; trying to conceive after stillbirth; telling people; unknown cause of stillbirth; and work after stillbirth
Stillbirth Collaborative Research Network (SCRN), 214–15
stillborn. *See* stillbirth
subsequent child, 42–44, 74, 147, 168–70; not a replacement for a stillborn baby, 34, 68, 73
subsequent pregnancy, xiv, 54, 61–63, 72, 100, 168–70; another loss during, 17, 74, 129; healing aspects of, 17; helps with moving on, 17; labor and delivery in a, 54, 62; medical management of, 192, 197; tests to request before a, 191–92; timing of, 190–91. *See also* anxiety during a subsequent pregnancy and trying to conceive after stillbirth
support group, 40, 41, 53–54, 125–33, 138, 166, 179; resistance to attending, 122, 128, 138
survivor guilt, 66–67

Tan, Meng Kiat, xix, 57–63, 246
telling people, 1–2, 3, 5, 16–17, 48–49, 68, 144. *See also* sharing your story; and living children, telling about the stillbirth
therapy after stillbirth, 129, 143, 146, 149, 181–83
Threads of Love, 178
time with the stillborn baby: stories of, 14–15, 20, 39, 73, 98, 104, 113; fear about spending, 122
triplets. *See* multiples
trying to conceive after stillbirth, 128, 190–92. *See also* subsequent pregnancy
twin-to-twin transfusion syndrome, 189

ultrasound: confirmation of death through, 14, 29–30, 42, 46, 72, 89, 97, 119–20, 122, 127, 136; use in monitoring subsequent pregnancy, 192, 195–97, 201–4, 208, 210–11
umbilical cord accidents: autopsy and, 213; common anomalies, 202; diagnosing, 188–89, 201; fetal behavior and, 201–2; monitoring, 202–4; preventing stillbirth due to, 201–4; recurrence risk, 192, 204; research involving, 188–89; stories of, 2, 8, 34, 135, 137, 148–49. *See also* Jason Collins and maternal blood pressure
umbilical cord function, 200–201
unexplained stillbirth. *See* unknown cause of stillbirth
unknown cause of stillbirth, 9–12, 46, 51, 129, 187; and anxiety, 200
Usher, Robert, 186

validation of your experience, 23–24, 105, 145–46, 175
vasa previa, 203
Villmer, Laura, xix, 95–101, 246
visitations. *See* signs from the baby
visual arts and grief, 41, 140, 148–49, 178–79; drawing of the baby, 107
volunteering, 55, 178–79

Walk to Remember, 74, 115, 175
Warland, Jane, 199, 205–6, 206, 209
"Where's your baby?" 1–2, 5, 144
Williams, Virginia, xviii, xxi, 1–5, 246–47
work after stillbirth, 15–17, 73, 105, 128, 145, 147; employer not granting enough time off from, 142; escape from sadness at, 40
worries about living children, 99
writing after stillbirth, xiii, 17, 50, 73, 130, 141–43, 177; prompts, 181–83

Yingst, Angie, xix, 45–50, 247

About the Contributors

Amy L. Abbey is the editor of *Journeys: Stories of Pregnancy after Loss* (Woven Word Press, 2006) and the owner of www.PregnancyJourneysAfterLoss.com. She has been a guest speaker at Winthrop University Hospital's Perinatal Bereavement Program since 2001. Abbey served on the planning committee for the First Candle/SIDS Alliance's second annual conference in 2005, which afforded her the opportunity to lobby in Washington, D.C., for continued funding for preventing SIDS and stillbirth. Abbey was honored as a Woman of Fortune by the Long Island Press (June 2006) and given the Woman of Distinction Award by New York Senate Assemblyman Bob Barra (14th Assembly District) in December 2007.

Janel C. Atlas is a freelance writer and editor whose work has appeared in various regional and national publications. Since her daughter's stillbirth, Atlas has written extensively about pregnancy and infant loss and spoken with many leading researchers in the field. She studied English literature at Messiah College in Pennsylvania and now lives in Delaware with her husband and daughters.

Nina Bennett, whose educational background is in psychology, is the author of *Forgotten Tears: A Grandmother's Journey through Grief* (Booklocker, Inc., 2005). She was a childbirth educator for nearly ten years and has worked in the HIV/AIDS field since the beginning of the epidemic. A frequently requested guest lecturer, Bennett presents workshops nationally on issues of perinatal bereavement and the grief of grandparents. Bennett is also a contributing author to Open to Hope, a bereavement website. Bennett served as the principal investigator of an IRB-approved research study looking at how grandparents incorporate perinatal loss into their family. Her articles and poetry have appeared in publications including *Philadelphia Stories*, *Pirene's Fountain*, *Mourning Sickness*, *The Broadkill Review*, *Slow Trains Literary Journal*, *Grief Digest*, *Different Kind of Parenting*, *M.I.S.S.ing Angels*, and *Living Well Journal*.

Joanne Cacciatore, specializes in counseling those affected by traumatic losses, most often the death of a child. She is board certified in bereavement trauma by the American Academy of Experts in Traumatic Stress and the National Center for Crisis Management. She is also board certified through the American Psychotherapy Association. Dr. Cacciatore founded the Center for Loss and Trauma/MISS Foundation, and since 1996 she has been working directly with families who experience the death of a child. She spearheaded and now directs the Certificate of Trauma and Bereavement graduate program at Arizona State University, where she is currently an assistant professor and researcher.

Marion J. Flores is the chief editor, web designer, and a journalist for www.newagevenus.com. She is an active mother of two special needs children. Prior to her children, Flores worked as an emergency medical technician. Flores has lived in New Jersey, Wisconsin, and Nevada and currently resides in Oregon. Flores's first novel is currently under agent review. She has been a foster parent to nearly a dozen abused, neglected, and abandoned children.

Ruth Fretts, MD, MPH, is an obstetrician gynecologist who currently practices in the Boston area at Harvard Vanguard Medical Associates and is an assistant professor at Harvard Medical School. She began her research on stillbirth during her residency at McGill University in Montreal in 1988–1992 with neonatologist Dr. Robert Usher. In 2002 she joined International Stillbirth Alliance (ISA), a not-for-profit group formed by parents. She was chair of their scientific committee until 2010; their international meetings bring parents and researchers together to tackle important issues including stillbirth awareness, advocacy, research, bereavement care, and prevention. She is the medical director for First Candle's Kicks Count! Campaign, which is designed to educate women about the importance of keeping track of fetal movement during pregnancy. She has published extensively on the topic of stillbirth including the *Technical Bulletin of Stillbirth* for the American College of Obstetrics and Gynecology. She lives in Brookline, Massachusetts, with her husband and three children.

Alan Goldenbach has been a staff writer for the *Washington Post* since 1999. His feature writing and investigative reporting have received awards from the Associated Press sports editors. He also authored *From the Ground Up*, an as-told-to autobiography of a boy born without legs who went on to become a standout high school wrestler (Sports Publishing, 2006). Goldenbach earned a BA in history from the University of Michigan. He can be reached at alangoldenbach@yahoo.com.

Rachel Graham lives in Manchester, England, with her husband and three children. She is an occupational therapist and works to design homes that are safe and accessible for children with disabilities. She is a volunteer for SANDS, a charity that supports bereaved parents after a baby death.

David Hlavsa heads the theatre arts department at Saint Martin's University in Lacey, Washington, where he has been teaching acting, directing, and playwriting since 1989. A recipient of the university's Outstanding Teaching Award, Hlavsa has twice served as faculty president. His article, "My First Son, A Pure Memory," was published in the "Modern Love" column of the *New York Times*. His latest play, *Pack of Lies*, has been widely produced. As an arts writer for the Seattle Repertory Theatre, he published more than a dozen articles and study guides on Goldoni, Feydeau, Lyle Kessler, Chekhov, Synge, Shakespeare, Pirandello, August Wilson, and others. Hlavsa has a BA in English/theatre from Princeton University and an MFA in directing from the University of Washington. He lives in Seattle with his wife and their son, Benjamin.

Sherokee Ilse continues her mission of mothering her living children and caring for and about bereaved parents around the world. She travels extensively, giving talks and seminars; writes articles and books; and recently began a consulting practice called Babies Remembered Consulting, working with hospitals, clinics, funeral homes, and churches in an effort to assess and improve their programs. Ilse, the author of many books, including *Empty Arms*, can be reached through her websites: www.babiesremembered.org or www.wintergreenpress.com.

Kara L. C. Jones, along with her husband, Hawk, cofounded KotaPress in 1999 after the stillbirth of their son Dakota. She is author of *Mrs. Duck and* *the Woman* and *Flash of Life* and is the lexicographer behind the *Dictionary of Loss*. As a grief and creativity coach, Jones founded the 1,000 Faces of Mother Henna project, facilitates workshops such as "The Hero's Journey" and "heART of Life and Death," and hosts creative explorations on both the Mother Henna and the KOTA blogs. Along with Dr. Joanne Cacciatore and Dr. John DeFrain, Jones has coauthored a series of articles exploring the effects of stillbirth. Their pieces have been featured in the *Ambiguous Loss Symposium*, *Journal of Family Social Work*, and *Marriage and Family Review*. Her website is www.motherhenna.com.

Kelley Krahling is a wife and mother. She has three living children in addition to her stillborn son. Krahling is an active volunteer in several nonprofit organizations and president of the PTA at her children's school. She maintains a blog in the stillbirth/neonatal/child loss community and is currently at work on her first book. She can be reached via e-mail at kelleykrahling@yahoo.com.

Monica Murphy LeMoine is a Highline Community College writing faculty member who lost her first son at 4 months' gestation and her second son to stillbirth at 32 weeks. She earned her master's in English at the University of Wisconsin, Milwaukee, and taught English as a Peace Corps volunteer in Uzbekistan. She is the founding editor of *Exhale*, an online literary magazine that focuses on miscarriage, stillbirth, infertility, and other childless-not-by-choice experiences. Her humorous memoir *Knocked Up, Knocked Down* was recently published by Catalyst Books. Murphy's work has been published in the magazines *Reality Mom*, *Hip Mama*, *KotaPress Compassion Journal*, and *Mamazine*. LeMoine has an infant son. She can be reached through her blog at http://knockedupknockeddown.blogspot.com.

Candy McVicar is the founder and executive director of Missing GRACE Foundation, an international support organization helping families on their journey through pregnancy and infant loss, infertility, and adoption. After the heartbreak of a failed domestic adoption, McVicar dealt with infertility and found that the support she needed was not readily available for these related but separate grief issues. She made a commitment to help others through the grief and pain she had known and to bring about awareness of these issues; she formed The Missing GRACE Foundation to aid individuals as they Grieve, Restore, Arise, Commemorate, and Educate. McVicar lectures across the country at hospitals, clinics, universities, churches, and conferences. She, her husband, Stephen, and daughters, Tatum and Talyah, live in the Twin Cities.

Tim Nelson wrote *A Father's Story—When a Baby Dies*, shortly after his daughter's stillbirth. It was one of the first perinatal loss support booklets written for men. More recently he wrote *A Guide for Fathers—When a Baby Dies* and coauthored *Couple Communication after a Baby Dies—Differing Perspectives*. He co-owns A Place to Remember, a grief publishing company that distributes resources for families and caregivers. Nelson is certified by the Grief Recovery Institute as a training specialist, and conducts outreach programs for those experiencing change and loss in their lives. He has spoken both nationally and internationally on topics of grief and loss. Nelson and his wife, Monica, have four living children. Nelson's blog can be found at http://fathersgrievinginfantloss.blogspot.com.

Jenell Williams Paris is professor of anthropology at Messiah College in Grantham, Pennsylvania. She has authored four books, including *Cultural Anthropology in Christian Perspective* (Baker Bookhouse, 2010) and a forthcoming book about sexual identity (InterVarsity Press, 2010). Her scholarly and popular articles have been published in journals and magazines including the *Los Angeles Times Online*, *The Christian Century*, *Christianity Today*, *Transforming Anthropology*, and *Gender, Place, and Culture*.

Suzanne Pullen is a communications instructor, lecturer, performer, and writer. The former journalist for the *San Francisco Chronicle* wrote two magazine articles, "Calling All Angels" and "Hope with a Heartbeat," about stillbirth and subsequent pregnancy, both of which received overwhelming responses from readers. "Calling All Angels" was a finalist for the Missouri Prize in Journalism. Pullen returned to academia to research the interactions between health care providers and bereaved parents and received her master's degree in communication studies from San Francisco State University in May 2010. In 2009, her paper "Giving Birth to Death" won a Top Paper award at the Western States Communications Association Convention, and she was named Galinson Scholar by the CSU trustees. In 2010, she debuted her new interactive play and workshop "He Was *Still* Born: How one mother delivered the gift of a lifetime and found the words that made a difference." Pullen is on the communications and parent advisory committees for the International Stillbirth Alliance, is a volunteer advocate with First Candle and First Breath, and also works with local bereavement groups. She plans to pursue her PhD in 2011. Pullen has one living son, Quinn.

Kathleen Skipper is a registered nurse, writer, lecturer, and mentor for the bereaved. She holds a BS in human services. She worked as a labor and delivery nurse for twenty-four years before founding Caring Arms, an in-hospital perinatal bereavement program, in 1990. She conducted perinatal bereavement conferences for physicians and staff on an ongoing basis. Besides facilitating five support groups, Skipper has provided one-on-one care for parents who chose to carry their babies with lethal anomalies. In addition to many articles, Skipper authored *A Rose Is God's Autograph*, a story about the loss of her two sons. She received the New York State Nurse of Distinction Award twice from her health care system and the C.A.R.E. Award from the Catholic Health System. Skipper continues to lecture and mentor on behalf of the bereaved. She has three living children.

Meng Kiat Tan's background is in art history. She has taught in colleges and worked in an art gallery. She currently homeschools her three daughters while working as a freelance writer and arts translator. She maintains two blogs, one a loose chronicle of their homeschooling life and the other about her meandering journey after her son Ferdinand's birth. Tan was one of the founding writers of *Glow in the Woods*, a group blog dedicated to providing voice and support to parents who have lost babies at various stages (www.glowinthewoods.com). She has lived in the United States (in Arizona) for nine years.

Laura Villmer is married to her wonderful husband, Charlie, and has three daughters. After spending two years studying at St. Cloud State University in Minnesota, she returned home to start her life with Charlie, and earned her bachelor's degree in communication from the University of Missouri, St. Louis in 2000. Always a sports enthusiast, Villmer began covering the local high school sports scene for the *Jefferson County Journal*, where she worked until she gave birth to her third daughter in 2006. After Madeline's stillbirth, Villmer began working from home. Villmer continues to do some freelance work and is currently at work on a book about her third pregnancy, focusing on her day-to-day challenges of pregnancy after the stillbirth.

Virginia Williams's publishing credits include working as a columnist for ClubMom.com, an online community with over two million members, contributing articles to the Absolute Write e-newsletter, the website WeddingChickie.com, and work as a Buzz Blogger for Prevention.com. Additionally, she has worked extensively as a PR and marketing copywriter and as a freelance writing consultant for several companies in the United States and England. Other writing credits include articles featured in regional parenting, travel, and business magazines. Prior to becoming a freelance writer and editor, Williams worked as a freelance proofreader and in-house copyeditor for Anness Publishing in London. She blogs about parenting after a loss at http://landofbrokenhearts.blogspot.com, and is currently at work on her first book.

Angie M. Yingst became a stay-at-home mother in 2007 after many years of working in a corporate marketing department as a writer, editor, and creative coordinator. Her poetry has been published in several print and online publications, including *Mothering Magazine*, *Literary Mama*, *Exhale Magazine*, and the now-defunct *In the Rearview*. Since the death of her second daughter in December 2008, Yingst has maintained a blog called Still Life with Circles (http://stilllifewithcircles.blogspot.com), dealing primarily with mothering and grief. Yingst is the editor of the website still life 365 (http://stilllife365.blogspot.com), which publishes pieces of art, poetry, music, or craft by grieving parents. When she is not writing, Yingst paints and illustrates mizuko jizo and other subjects dealing with baby loss, pregnancy, and parenting at her Etsy shop. Yingst holds a bachelor's degree in comparative religion from Temple University.